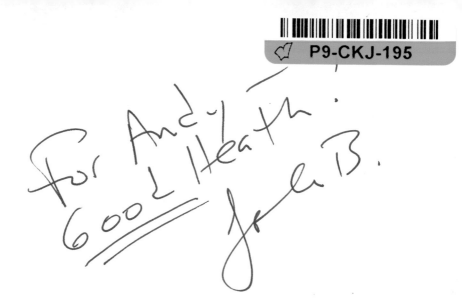

For Andy Heath.
Good Heath
John B.

The Santa Barbara Diet

by
John Bishop

First Edition

Printed by Rincon Press
P.O Box 1370, Wilson, Wyoming
Publisher's Cataloging-in-Publication
(Provided by Quality Books, Inc.)

Bishop, John, 1951-
    The Santa Barbara Diet / by John Bishop. -- 1st ed.
    p. cm.
    Includes bibliographical references and index.
    ISBN-13: 978-0-9795616-3-4 (softcover)
    ISBN-10: 0-9795616-3-9 (softcover)

    1. Health. 2. Nutrition.   I. Title.

RA776.9.B57 2007   613

QBI07-600133

Dedication

This book is dedicated to Duke Paoa Kahanamoku, the first Hawaiian Olympian, The Father of Modern Surfing, and Hawaii's Aloha Ambassador to the World.

Duke lived the spirit that Hawaiian poet Pilahi Paki wrote about:

A — *Akahai: kindness, expressed with tenderness*
L — *Lakahi: unity, expressed with harmony*
O — *Oluolu: agreeable, expressed with pleasantness*
H — *Haahaa: humility, expressed with modesty*
A — *Ahonui: patience, expressed with perseverance*

Duke won his first Gold Medal at age 22 in Stockholm Sweden in 1912. He was 42 years old when he competed in his last Olympic events. He won more than Gold Medals—he won the hearts of people all over the world for his grace in the water, good humor, and sportsmanship.....

His Aloha lives on....

The Santa Barbara Diet
by
John Bishop

TABLE OF CONTENTS

NOTE FROM THE AUTHOR

You are holding in your hands a health and nutrition book unlike any other you've ever read. It's my sincere wish that *The Santa Barbara Diet* makes an enormous change in your life.

In this book, I've tried to make important medical and scientific health information easy and accessible, so you can avoid being conned by the profit-motivated agendas of big business, politics, and modern medicine. Knowledge is power, and being forewarned leaves you forearmed and empowered, especially when it comes to the sacred subject of your own personal good health.

My audience is primarily the 80 million baby boomers I grew up with, but people of all ages and locales can benefit from the information I present. My message is simple: If you're an American, you've spent your life as a human lab rat in a gigantic, uncontrolled dietary experiment that evidence now shows has failed. The results of this experiment, performed on you without your consent or knowledge, demonstrate conclusively that the American diet is toxic for your health, and the primary cause of both cancer and heart disease.

I chose to call my first book *The Santa Barbara Diet* to honor the beautiful city I fell in love with when I moved here from the Midwest with my family in 1964. To me, Santa Barbara will always represent a certain state of mind that's an awareness of how life should be: healthful, energetic, and enjoyable. Somehow I always feel more in tune with what life's all about when I'm in Santa Barbara. Perhaps it's the cosmic duality of the clear light and the cold foggy days, or the contrast between the uplifted mountain ranges and the deep blue waters of the Pacific Ocean. For me, Santa Barbara has always been a place of stunning contrast and natural beauty. With so much to offer every day, the Santa Barbara lifestyle allows you to either seize the day or simply kick back and enjoy it.

This dual nature of the Santa Barbara experience, in the natural setting and the range of lifestyles, is reflected in *The Santa Barbara Diet* by a major theme, which is that there are always two sides to every coin. It is not the food we eat that makes us unhealthy, but the food we are sold and what has been done to it in the interests of profit and business. You will be reading of many foods you thought were "taboo" for one reason or another, but in truth are only off the healthy list because of how they are produced and/or processed.

I wrote this book from my personal experiences as I journeyed on the path of what it takes to be a healthy human being. My perspective is unique—I'm not a doctor, I'm not trying to sell you vitamins or heart surgery, and I'm not an academic. I'm just an average person who found out what you and I need to do to be healthy by asking questions.

Here are some of the questions that forced me to keep digging deeper as I researched this book:

✓ Why do Americans, who consume more dairy products than almost anyone, have some of the world's highest rates of osteoporosis?

✓ What caused the heart disease epidemic in America that started in the 1920s and peaked in 1968?

✓ Why have heart disease rates fallen sharply since 1968?

✓ Why would a recent ten year study (Finnish-Harvard study) show that taking only 700 milligrams of vitamin C daily reduces the incidence of heart disease by over 25%?

✓ Why do animals almost never get heart disease?

✓ Why does eating seafood twice a week drop the rate of heart disease by over 30%?

✓ Why does eating one ounce of nuts twice a week reduce heart disease by 30%?

✓ Why do dieters in America often lose their hair or have thinning hair when they diet?

In the research I did, I was shocked to find out that Americans are spending over twice as much per capita on health care as any other country, yet according to the World Health Organization, we're in 37th place for overall health. One of the main reasons, I discovered, is because the practice of medicine has been a *for profit* business in America ever since the 1970s. Much of the current health crisis also involves the lack of representation in Washington, D.C. advocating for the health of the average citizen.

A great deal of what I learned came from actions taken by government regulators in countries like the U.K., Switzerland, Sweden, Germany and Japan. These countries aren't exactly health utopias either, but at least the interests of their citizens haven't been so blatantly sold down the river as they have in America.

Obviously, one can't talk about changing our country's medical system without getting lawyers out of the doctors' pockets. America is now a country run by and for the benefit of lawyers, and at both a state and national level, over half of our legislators are lawyers. Here are a few steps I believe are urgently needed to reform medical care in the U.S. to impact our national state of health:

- ✓ Adopt a single-payer national health care system.
- ✓ The loser pays the winner's costs in all lawsuits.
- ✓ Go back to the system used in England and Canada and stop letting lawyers pick juries. Seat the first 12 qualified people.
- ✓ Cap all pain and suffering awards at $1 million.
- ✓ Ban all advertising on TV, the Internet, and print media for prescription drugs.

In *The Santa Barbara Diet*, you will learn more about some of the largest frauds I've uncovered regarding the manufacture and sale of cholesterol lowering drugs, surgical treatments for heart disease, extensive use of chemotherapy, marketing of industrial dairy products, and the false claims that soy products are good for your heart.

It's too bad the late George Orwell, author of *1984* and *Animal Farm*, isn't around to help me make some pithy comments on the shenanigans of the corporate sharks, disgraced presidents worrying about their legacy, and the corruption of democracy that I've uncovered in my research. What was truly surprising in my discoveries is how inexpensive my recommendations are and how easy it is to improve your health. I was shocked to learn that over 75% of all medical expenditures in the U.S. involve heart disease, obesity and diabetes, all conditions that can be treated naturally and are completely preventable.

I urge you to use the healthy living practices found in this book. I hope they change your life as they did mine.....

To your good health!

John Bishop

July 7th, 2007

CHAPTER ONE

How To Be A Healthy Human Being

Like most people, I'm sure you have struggled through the many contradictory theories about diet, health, nutrition, and medical advice that's been available to the public over the last 30 or so years. If those messages seemed confusing, I'm sure the little data bytes of information you've received via the Internet, TV, and TV advertising in recent years has only made you more confused.

When I started writing this book about how to be healthy, I realized I was like a ship's navigator in the 1600s before the invention of the astrolabe or the sextant. How would you like to navigate a ship in perilous seas near rocky coasts with no good method to establish your longitude or to have a good fix on your location? When it comes to steering a course to avoid cancer or heart disease, you want to have more to go on than relying upon a navigator (your local doctor) who wants you to trust his sense of which way the wind is blowing, or his "instincts" of the direction the current is carrying you.

This is a science-based book, and I'm giving you information that takes you from relying upon the advice of your local ship pilot and gives you the equivalent of a Globally Positioned Satellite (GPS), to help you steer a course to the Land of Good Health. If you're an average citizen, what you don't know is that most of your ailments can be avoided. Most disease in America happens by choice—not chance. It's up to you to put your hand upon the tiller, make the right choices, and steer yourself away from the perilous medical shoals so many of us drift onto by not choosing to live a healthy life. Choice—*not chance*—should rule your life!

Disease and Your Diet

Most disease in America has dietary origins, and most cancer and heart disease is predictable, preventable, and highly avoidable. I've been skeptical of many things in my lifetime here in America, but even I was surprised by what I discovered in researching this book. I'm writing specifically for Americans, but this message applies to people all over the world whose health has been influenced by the practices of modern agriculture, commerce, and medicine.

One of the things I'm going to give you in *The Santa Barbara Diet* is simple vitamin formulas that can prevent and reverse heart disease. My health recommendations are incredibly cheap and harmless compared to the complex, expensive technological fixes offered by modern medicine. Always keep this in mind; most people are born with a healthy body. It's what you *do* to your body that creates ill health. One hundred years ago Americans were some of the healthiest people in the world. How could we spend twice as much as any other country on health care and be so unhealthy? My question is this: *Why shouldn't Americans be the healthiest and happiest people in the world?*

Some of what you find in this book might be controversial, but what I'm giving you is really a dose of old-time common sense. Here are the facts: As recently as 70 or 80 years ago, very few Americans had heart disease or cancer. As sickly, obese, and unhealthy as Americans are today—it's hard to imagine how much healthier Americans were in 1920. Most people when presented with this information are in denial and want to continue believing cancer or heart disease was common back then. *It just wasn't reported or they didn't have good statistics or good doctors back then*, is what even educated people believe. Sorry folks, the facts go like this: Cancer and heart disease were extremely rare in America at the beginning of the 20th century.

We didn't lack for competent medical observers back in 1920—it's just that back then, very few people in the prime of life died of heart disease and cancer. I'm not saying these diseases didn't exist, but they were primarily diseases of old age, as they should be now. The first recorded myocardial infarction (heart attack) wasn't noted in medical journals until 1912. What has developed in the last hundred years is an unprecedented epidemic of bad health caused primarily by the defective foods Americans eat.

For the majority of us, it isn't our genes or some mysterious X factor causing cancer or heart disease—it's our defective food choices and our diet lacking in vital nutrients that causes disease. Eating a diet loaded with toxic substances—refined sugars, high fructose corn syrups, faux sugars, soy proteins, hydrogenated oils, oxidized cholesterols, vitamin and mineral deficient canned and processed foods, pasteurized milks and cheeses, and meats loaded with hormones and antibiotics—has been decisively proven by a one hundred year experiment to be toxic to human beings. That experiment has failed. And these are the sort of products and life styles that American agri-business and commerce exports to the rest of the world?

Most diseases have dietary origins, yet our society spends billions of dollars looking for "cures" for disease, when disease can be drastically reduced by prevention. Of course, one should never forget there are no guarantees in this life, and bad things can and do happen to good people. I'm not guaranteeing perfect outcomes from eating and living right—but your personal choices can greatly improve your chances of living a long and healthy life. I can say confidently, there's more information in this book to help you find your way through the smoke screens of disinformation being put out by Big Pharma, the Medical Industrial Complex, and the FDA than any other health book ever published. I realize I'm promising you a lot in the last sentence, but as Muhammad Ali said back in the Roaring Sixties—*It ain't bragging, if you can back it up!*

Sadly, we live in the sort of world where if you want to do something to increase your country's gross national product, few things you could do would have the same effect as developing heart disease or cancer. If you were so unfortunate as to get cancer, you might need as much as $1 million worth of medical treatment.

This reminds me of what happened near the incredibly beautiful city of Hue in Vietnam in January of 1968, during what we Americans call the Tet Offensive. When Hue was seized by the Viet Cong, American military forces unleashed a hellish bombardment of artillery shells and bombing, after which one American soldier was quoted as saying, "We had to destroy the city to save it." One of the largest religious complexes ever built in Asia was reduced to rubble, and today only a few buildings survive. This is a good analogy for the immaculate temple of your body and what your body would be like if you survived heart disease and cancer treatments. A lot of modern medicine's treatments are worse than the disease.

I realize my message might be controversial compared to the

simple "truths" delivered to you by the Medical Establishment or by the cheery representatives of the pharmaceutical industry, otherwise known as Big Pharma. My message of how to be a healthy human being involves more than being a true believer of simplistic verities. Jingoism might play well in short sound bites on Fox News, but it doesn't put a healthy glow in your cheeks or make you happy or healthy. When Albert Einstein was a young boy, he saw the soldiers of what would become Nazi Germany goose-stepping through the streets, and he made his parents promise him they would never make him be a soldier. The lesson to be learned from what Einstein thought as a child is a simple one—*Think for yourself.*

Of course, there are a lot of other factors involved in staying healthy than your diet. Never forget we live in a world where over 100 million human beings died fighting wars in the last century. For the sake of your own good mental health: *Practice forgiveness.* Violence begets violence…and to be a healthy human being, you need to reject the idea of getting even.

There are some who might criticize me for leaving out the spiritual side of health and healing and good health. I certainly didn't intend to leave it out—I just left that up to you. After all, that's between you and the Great Spirit. As one of America's greatest poets once said: *To each his own—it's all unknown….*

As I've said, this is a science-based book, and we all live in a world created by both the fruits and the detritus of modern science. Pick and choose—I encourage you to make wise choices. I do believe that the choice before us all is best stated by Stewart Brand, founder of the *Whole Earth Catalogue*: "We are as Gods—and we damn well better get good at it, quick!"

If there's anything controversial in writing about choosing good health, the discussion should include the billions of dollars of profit that is made by American agri-business, the pharmaceutical industry, and the medical/industrial complex every year by keeping you ignorant of what you need to do to be a healthy human being. As I'm writing this, I'm keenly aware that my stepping between large corporations and their perceived *right to profit* from mass marketing defective products isn't going to make them happy. Growth for the sake of growth is, and always has been, one of the cornerstones of American capitalism.

However, growth for the sake of growth is also the ideology of the cancer cell. My own personal experience tells me that these large corporations will do all they can to discredit messages that might upset their golden applecart. All I can say is: *Don't shoot the messenger! Shoot the message……*

It is my hope that this book will teach you healthy habits to help you avoid being a statistic in America's national epidemic of bad health. Unlike most of the people who write health and nutrition books, I'm not a salesman trying to sell you a line of vitamins (Atkins Diet) or a heart surgeon (South Beach Diet) trying to make you lose weight or give you canned, formulaic inaccurate advice on your diet.

My Own Health Story

After I turned 50 in 2001, I had a few small health problems, and in the process of figuring them out, I lost a considerable amount of faith in the medical system. The more I tried to fix my own minor health problems and figure out what I should do, the more I became confused. I slowly realized that many of the so-called medical expert's opinions contradicted each other, and that you really were on your own in figuring the best path to take. *The Santa Barbara Diet* is the story of my journey down that path.

My most pressing problem in 2001 was that my feet had started swelling near the joints in my toes, the result of hiking on a trail in Santa Barbara three or four years earlier. Because of this, it started being difficult to wear shoes when I was physically active. I'd been able to ignore or minimize this problem for a few years until I had good health insurance. It was then that I decided to be pro-active and do something about it.

I visited a local orthopedic surgeon with good credentials, and he did an operation on one of my feet to correct what he said was a "bone spur." Within a month's time, I realized the operation he had done was useless and hadn't fixed the problem.

A year later, through word of mouth, I found a doctor in a nearby city who was an expert in foot surgery. When I saw him, I discovered the swelling was caused by friction from the collagen wearing out in the joints of my big toes. Upon examination with X-rays, this was extremely obvious.

So, I was only 50 and I'd worn out the cartilage in both of my toe joints. I'd been physically active as a skier and hiker and had worked as a commercial diver for 14 years—but had that been enough activity to wear out my cartilage? At that time, I accepted the diagnosis without questioning why this had happened. However, this seemed somewhat strange to me, as I was only 50 years old.

Back then, I was still a believer in traditional medical advice, so I had a successful surgery by an experienced and capable specialist, who, unlike the previous orthopedic surgeon that had operated on my foot to correct the "bone spur," actually knew what he was doing. I had one of the toe joints fused and had a specialized procedure on the other one to give me more years before it, too, I was told, would need to be fused.

The surgery was successful—but then my feet didn't heal. I ended up spending 14 weeks on crutches during both a Jackson Hole winter and a month-long trip to Asia which had been planned before the surgery. The next question was: *Why didn't my feet heal?*

The answer I discovered was that the healing process was not complete until two years later when I starting taking large doses of vitamin C. The sensations of discomfort that lingered on after the surgery disappeared within a few weeks of taking 4,000 to 5,000 milligrams of vitamin C daily. I also began to wonder if the problem caused by wearing out the collagen in my toe joints might have been avoided if I'd been taking the amounts of vitamin C my body needed, in the first place.

Your body can't manufacture a single molecule of vitamin C, I discovered, and if you're physically active and subjected to stress, you'll need more than normal amounts of vitamin C. Vitamin C is essential for healing from any surgery, and optimum amounts of it are critical in your body's manufacture of collagen—the connective tissue holding your body together.

I should mention here my family history is probably similar to many people's—we have a history of cancer. My father died in his early 50s from a brain tumor, and one of my uncles also died of bladder cancer. My mother recently survived breast cancer surgery while in her late 70s, and is now in good health. Her breast cancer was diagnosed and treated with competent medical procedures, yet it was an iatrogenic (doctor-caused) disease. Her cancerous breast tumors were a common side-effect of the hormonal drug Premarin she took for 23 years. So— common medical practices caused the cancer. Then they fixed it. Does this make sense to you? Somehow, it seems to me like buying fake diamonds with counterfeit money....

Actually, my medical problems turned out to be a blessing in disguise, because they forced me to discover what I need to know to live a long and healthy life. I started reading many health books and became obsessed with figuring it all out. The more I read, the more I realized that the "experts" often don't agree, and many medical theories that treatments are based upon are of questionable veracity.

We've Been Fooled Before

Being an American, I'd walked down the path of trusting the experts before, and it's a path I've learned can be dangerous to your health and well being. I'm keenly aware I've grown up in a country where many of our government's follies and frauds, such as open air nuclear testing, the Vietnam War, the War on Drugs, and the War on Terrorism have been blandly accepted by the general public. As the truth came out, more and more gradually came to see open air nuclear testing and the Vietnam War as disastrous, failed policies—yet the War on Drugs and the War on Terrorism are still rolling forward. How serious could the War on Terrorism be, when at the beginning of 2007, according to a report on the NBC Evening News, almost six years after September 11th, the FBI has only 33 agents of 12,000 that speak Arabic?

What I discovered in writing this book is that much of the medical advice and practices in America are as wrong and as dangerous to your good health as some of the other immense frauds our system of governance and culture have encouraged during my lifetime.

In the 1950s, while we were eating our Sugar Smacks and playing with Hula Hoops, the U.S. Government maintained open air nuclear testing was harmless. Tests showed radiation caused "hybrid vigor" in fruit flies and that genetic mutations were good for you. Young Americans in the Armed Forces were used as human guinea pigs and as "observers" of open air nuclear bomb tests without being given any protective gear. The powers that be also stated nuclear power was "safe" and "harmless," and using nuclear power would make electricity so cheap it would be "almost free."

The intervention of the United States in a civil war in Vietnam was also presented as "necessary" and "urgent" to end attempts by communists to dominate the world. Ultimately, this insane and stupid war ended in 1975 with one of smallest and poorest countries in the world defeating the U.S.A.

As I found from the research I did for *The Santa Barbara Diet,* if you follow the money trail—you'll discover a great deal of what has been represented as reasonable and sensible practices are a veritable grab bag of lies. I never imagined that what you need to do to live a healthy life could be so drastically different from the widely accepted practices of modern medicine, agriculture and pharmacology. I happened to learn a great deal about our government's monumental failed programs as I grew up—yet I didn't imagine the story of how to have good health would be so similar.

I wouldn't want anyone to think from what I'm saying that I'm anti-American. Nothing could be further from the truth. I'm proud to be an American, but my vision of America might be a little different than most. My heroes have always been Americans—who wouldn't want to meet George Washington, Crazy Horse, Sitting Bull, John James Audubon, Touch the Clouds, Walt Whitman, Chief Joseph, Winslow Homer, Herman Melville, Black Elk, Thomas Edison, Ishi, Charlie Russell, Duke Kahanamoku, Bessie Smith, Jack Johnson, Luther Burbank, Jelly Roll Morton, Woody Guthrie, Billy Holliday, Charles Lindbergh, Wovoka, Louie Armstrong, John Steinbeck, Robert Johnson, Isadora Duncan, Charley Parker, Howard Hughes, Chuck Berry, Captain Trips, Rosa Parks, Linus Pauling, Marilyn Monroe, Ernest Hemingway, John Kennedy, Ken Kesey, Andrew Wyeth, Stevie Wonder, Muhammad Ali, T.C. Cannon, Geena Davis or Bob Dylan?

Choosing to walk a healthy path in life will help you avoid most of the calamities befalling those who go through life plowing a field like a mule with blinders on. Is it really any fun plowing that field and never looking up and seeing what the clouds and the sky look like? In the world's most capitalistic society, if you don't think for yourself—others will think for you—and you might wind up being a pawn in their game.

Before I figured out what you and I need to do to have good health, I always wondered why so many people in America had osteoporosis. How could you get osteoporosis when we Americans eat more calcium from dairy products than almost any country in the world? Doesn't calcium make strong bones? I also wondered why so many Americans get heart attacks and cancer when poor people in countries like the Philippines, Thailand, and rural China don't. And why was cancer and heart disease almost unknown in primitive populations?

I make my point about open air nuclear testing and the Vietnam War because I wanted to encourage you to keep an open mind when I expose many of the reasons why Americans are now some of the unhealthiest people in the world. We've been fooled before—and I'm giving you the information you need to keep the wool from being pulled over your eyes.

I believe I'm the first health writer to pull it all together and give you the big picture on how defective our agriculture practices, medical techniques, and pharmacology is in America. Don't despair though—the news is good! You can opt out of most of America's disease epidemic by changing your diet and your health practices.

Two Sides of the Same Coin

Understanding the duality about the information we have—how it is both correct and not correct—is an important theme that comes up often in this book. For example, a food may be healthy, but the way it is processed is not. The same applies for any procedure or theory—it's sound until you start messing with it. Then you begin to see that there are two sides to the same coin.

In the next chapter, you will see how the cholesterol explanation for heart disease fits that duality. I'm going to explain cholesterol to you in a different way than it's ever been explained before. It's simple and logical, and what I'm saying covers the facts much better than widely accepted unproven theories that are being fraudulently used to sell you billions of dollars of medicine annually under the guise of lowering your *bad* cholesterol. Obviously, the topic is much more complicated than just calling cholesterol *good* or *bad*. Your ignorance is leading you right into the warm embrace of America's big pharmaceutical companies. Ignorance is not bliss!

Duality is what the sugar story is all about, too. Honey and maple syrup are nutritious and good for you, yet refined sugar is toxic for your health. Refined sugar isn't a food—it's an anti-nutrient. And *high fructose corn syrup* is even worse. In many studies, it fattens laboratory rats up in record time. Why wouldn't it do the same for you? And, of course, sugar substitutes, like the neuro-toxin *aspartame,* are terrible for your good health, and natural sugar substitutes, like the herbal sweetener *stevia,* are completely harmless.

Processed, homogenized, pasteurized milk from factory cows isn't good for you, and raw, certified milk and cheeses from cows fed on grass are some of the best foods you can eat. Soy products are good for you too, but only when consumed in the traditional ways Asians eat them, in very small amounts and fermented for long periods of time. Soy products are a health hazard when consumed in the ways American agri-business serves them to misinformed vegetarians and vegans. Industrial salt is bad for you—over 95% of salt doesn't come from the shaker but is in processed foods—but healthy sea salt is good for you. Natural cholesterol from high quality sources, such as saturated fats from grass-fed, organic beef and buffalo, or coconut oil are very good for you. But oxidized cholesterols from polyunsaturated vegetable oils or hydrogenated soybean oils are toxic.

If you've never heard this message before, bear with me: All of these topics are explained in depth in the chapters that follow. Much of what I'm telling you might contradict the health messages you've heard most of your life, but it's time you started thinking for yourself and not being a victim of commercial propaganda. Basically, what I'm telling you is the bare-bones story of what you need to learn to drop your name off the roster of All-American victims of our National Bad Health Program. You deserve good health! It's your birthright to be a healthy, happy, disease-free human being.

Where's The Food?

The first step on your journey to good health is a stroll through your average American supermarket, where you will see that most of the "food"' on the shelves isn't really food. When I walk down the aisles of the average supermarket, I'm often reminded of the story told by social workers in the 1970s who helped re-settle Hmong tribal people from Laos into the suburbs of Minneapolis. Almost all of the Hmong spoke little or no English, but they enjoyed their supermarket tour immensely. They were fascinated by the cornucopia of brightly colored boxes, tins, and containers on the endless shelves. After getting a complete tour, one of the social workers had a translator ask if they had any questions. The Hmong seemed a little puzzled, and finally one of them asked, "Where's the food?"

The Hmong could understand the meat, vegetable and seafood section—but the rest of the American supermarket was a mystery. Was it really "food" in those containers, cans and boxes? I'm telling you this, because we need to start living like those Hmong tribal people from the distant hills of Southeast Asia and stop buying America's toxic, dysfunctional food products. Real food is food that's alive and has power and strength in it, food like most of the world eats—beans, peas, fruits, grains, vegetables, meats, and cheeses.

Let's stop for a moment and come on a tour of the average supermarket with me.....

Our first stop is the OXIDIZED CHOLESTEROLS department. I'm referring to the section where all of those polyunsaturated vegetable oils are being sold. Over 80% of your soybean and cheap cottonseed oils are hydrogenated for long shelf life. All of these oils are cheap industrial products and despite the hydrogenation process, are usually rancid. Because of this, all cooking oils should be stored carefully, bottled in dark bottles, and refrigerated. Does this handling resemble anything you're looking at in the oil section of your local supermarket?

Next stop is the WHITE BREAD department. It is true what those health food kooks said in the '60s and '70s—*The whiter the bread, the quicker you're dead.* You should think of white breads in the same way you think of candy. Eating as little as possible of foods containing bleached white flour is some of the best healthy living advice you've ever received. If you don't like whole grain food products, then you should avoid eating bread. The way most modern breads are made with bleached, refined flour, bread shouldn't be thought of as food. It's a machine-made product with little or no nutritional value. Pan Bimbo and Wonder Bread are the extreme spectrum of the bread zone. I'm not sure it's even a good idea feeding them to the sea gulls or pigeons. It's horrifying that some people feed children these ersatz foods.

I'd send you over to the SUGAR department, but unfortunately, due to the ubiquity of modern food processing, sugar is in almost every processed food in the store! And sugar's evil twin, *high fructose corn syrup* (HFCS), is lurking in most foods in the store. In a later chapter, I'll explain how HFCS is the secret sugar, the one that works overtime at making you fat.

One item that dominates in the ubiquitous SUGAR department is SODA POP, a "food" that is actually an incredible profit sector for large corporations such as PepsiCo and Coca-Cola. Soda pop is the sugar delivery vehicle that's the equivalent of a hypodermic needle for a drug addict. It's amazing that complacent consumers have sucked down these sugary beverages for so long. One of the unusual things about Coca-Cola and Pepsi products is their content of phosphoric acid which gives them a pH close to vinegar. However, the high sugar content masks this acidity. There's a good reason why they call them *soft* drinks—they'll make your bones go soft, if you drink too many of them!

Let me remind you again: sugar isn't a food—it's an anti-nutrient. This is probably the highest profit section of the supermarket for food marketers. However, the expenses of advertising to keep you thinking *It's the Real Thing!* or that *Things go Better with Coke* is starting to cut into their profits. Also, fighting off the government regulators beginning to zero in on this scam is starting to cost more than it used to. And the payola to schools getting *pouring rights* is beginning to be noticed by school districts where some pesky parents are getting pro-active about the health of their chubby kids who drink these sugary beverages.

Next stop is the CANNED FOODS section. This is another section where consumers shop who don't care much about how long they live. Canning vegetables strips away 45 to 80% of vitamins and minerals. And you expect to be a healthy human being eating this stuff?

And of course, the huge PROCESSED FOODS section of the supermarket is where you find the pastas made from refined bleached flours, the potato chips, crackers and so on. Most of these products have had 75 to 90% of their vitamins and minerals removed in their processing and manufacturing.

Then we come to the BREAKFAST CEREALS section. The real

truth about these highly advertised products is that when it comes to nutrition, they are seriously defective foods. Given their high sugar content, their hydrogenated oils, and chemicals added for taste, you might be better off eating the cardboard box and throwing away the cereal!

Being skeptical about your standard American food choices at the supermarket is a good place to start to be a healthy human being. The most important thing you can do to change your health is to understand that most of the dietary information you've received is questionable, at best.

My Top Ten Recommendations

I realize that many of you who are reading this book are overweight and would like to lose excess weight permanently. At the same time, I also recognize that you are malnourished because of a critical deficit of vitamins and minerals in the American diet. I'm going to give you a quick overview of what to do to make sure you have adequate nutrition in your diet before you attempt to lose weight. (Later, in Chapter 9, I'll show you how to use time-honored techniques like nutritionally fortified fasting to lose the weight.)

Here are my Top Ten Recommendations—if you do nothing else but follow these, you will have improved your chances of living a healthy life and succeeding at losing excess weight permanently. You may have other nutritional or medical needs, but these are good, all purpose programs for most people. As always, modify them for your own specific needs.

TOP TEN RECOMMENDATIONS FOR HEALTH AND WEIGHT LOSS

EAT MORE SATURATED FATS. Contrary to what you've been told all your life—saturated fats, such as fat on meat, chicken skin, butter, beef tallow, lard and coconut oil are excellent for your good health. There are good reasons why people all over the world have always prized high quality fats. Recent studies show that for calcium to be effectively utilized in our bones, at least 50% of dietary fats consumed should be saturated fats. Your body needs healthy and nutritious saturated fats, and not eating them creates food cravings, mood swings, dietary imbalances, and cravings for both sugar and fats. All your life, you've been told to eat lean meats by the dietary experts, yet Native Americans have known for centuries you cannot sustain life by eating animals that don't have fat reserves. Some of the early explorers of North America who didn't know this, almost starved to death trying to live on lean meat from animals without fat reserves killed in early spring or summer. In all cultures, people have always valued fat as a food, because it represents the highest amount of caloric intensity. And fat tastes good! After, the last Ice Age, our primitive ancestors quickly settled the far northern edges of the receding ice in Scandinavia and Canada as early as 11,000 B.C., because by killing animals living in cold climates, they obtained the largest amount of fat available with the least amount of effort. They were the venture capitalists of their era!

GO NATURAL, EAT REAL FOODS. Eat as much organic foods as you can afford. Eat a healthy amount of raw foods compared to your intake of processed and cooked foods. However, it isn't natural for humans to eat a diet of entirely raw foods, as some health experts would have you believe. Some cooked foods actually have higher vitamin and mineral contents than uncooked foods and some are barely edible without cooking. Also eating butter, avocados, olive oil or coconut oil with vegetables greatly increases your absorption of vitamins and minerals. Enzymes are also an important part of a healthy diet and are only found in live and unprocessed foods, such as raw milk, cheeses made from raw milk, juices that aren't pasteurized, uncooked fruits, raw unprocessed honey, figs, apples, bananas, sprouts and nuts and grains. Eating foods containing enzymes is believed by many experts, to be one of the best things you can do to improve your health and physical vitality.

EAT LESS SUGAR. Eating less than 50 pounds of sugar annually is critical to your good health.

TAKE MULTIPLE AND B VITAMINS. Make sure you take a good multiple vitamin and adequate amounts of B6, B12, and folic acid, and vitamin E from natural sources to help prevent heart disease. The primary cause of heart disease is chronic vitamin and mineral deficiencies. Heart disease is an inflammatory disease that has little to do your dietary cholesterol intake.

TAKE VITAMIN C. Your body cannot produce a single molecule of vitamin C and you need to make sure you take adequate amounts—at least 2,000 milligrams daily for the rest of your life.

TAKE MAGNESIUM. Making sure you have adequate amounts of magnesium both in your diet and in dietary supplements is critical to the health of your heart. Between 60 and 80% of All Americans are seriously deficient in magnesium. It's a critical factor in both osteoporosis and heart disease. Why risk your good health and lovely bones by not taking magnesium?

TAKE A DOSE OF COD LIVER OIL EVERY DAY. Lemon flavored is best.

TAKING A TABLESPOON OF BREWER'S YEAST DAILY. Brewer's yeast has strongly synergistic effects when it is combined with vitamin C for reducing the incidence of colds. It is available in bulk at your local health food store. In almost ten years of doing this, I have reduced my incidence of colds to almost zero.

TAKE AS FEW PRESCRIPTION DRUGS AND ANTIBIOTICS AS POSSIBLE. About antibiotics: Women who are heavy users of antibiotics have much higher rates of breast cancer than control groups. After taking antibiotics, you should always take a round of pro-biotic yoghurts (available at your local health food store) to help restore the natural flora and fauna in your intestines.

EAT AND COOK WITH COCONUT OIL. Adding coconut oil to your diet is one of the best health practices you will ever do. It is the healthiest saturated fat, as it is metabolized quicker than other saturated fats. The countries with the highest coconut oil consumption, the Philippines and Thailand, have the lowest cancer rates in the world. It's also good for your heart.

CHAPTER TWO

Eat Your Cholesterol— It's Good For You!

I started out thinking that because I'd grown up in Santa Barbara in the '60s and '70s, I knew a lot about natural foods and what was good for you. You can imagine my surprise as I did my research and much of what I believed about food, diet, and health got systematically shredded.

Little did I know what a complicated journey I was embarking on, trying to figure out the many conflicting opinions in the field of health and nutrition. Looking back now, I realize what you have to do to be a healthy human being isn't that complicated. I'm happy I've learned what it takes to be healthy, and I'm glad I can share this information with you.

I have to admit, however, it was a real struggle writing *The Santa Barbara Diet*. When I started, I was naïve enough to take seriously the advice of my many predecessors in the diet field. Following their advice, I painted myself into a lot of illogical corners, before I realized most of the experts were, at best, only about 50% right.

I was 52 when I began writing *The Santa Barbara Diet*, and my first step on the journey to becoming a healthy human being was to get my cholesterol levels tested. Like everyone else, I believed that the most important thing to do was test cholesterol to determine my risk of heart disease. After all, who would want to have heart surgery, if it could be avoided?

The thought of having open heart surgery was as attractive to me as being dragged up the steps of an Aztec temple and having my chest cut open with an obsidian dagger to be offered up as a sacrifice to the Sun Gods. We still do sacrifices here in America, but the victims now are mostly sacrificed not to make the sun come up, but to keep the wheels of commerce turning. More about that, later.....

On a different note, I once wandered down into the reserved parking lot at Cottage Hospital in Santa Barbara and couldn't help but notice the cars heart surgeons drive. It's ironic that the men who dress in the white coats prefer the color black for their BMW's, Lexus's, and Infiniti's. Those guys drive some expensive cars! And pardon my sexism, but this heart surgery business is mostly a male dominated business, just like the temple priest cults in the days of the Aztecs. I wouldn't be surprised if the behavior and bedside manner of the Aztec temple priests and the attitudes and opinions of your local heart surgeons didn't have a great deal in common. Frankly, their technological jargon is about as comprehensible as the chants of the temple priests in Aztec days. *Just lay back and relax—we'll take care of everything for you. We're going to make life better for you....*

One purpose of this book is to inform you about how you can avoid high-tech medical treatments by using foods and vitamins as your medicines. I have a simple belief that science and technology exist to serve us, rather than us existing to be served up as victims on the altars of Technology and Big Business.

The Cholesterol Dogma

One of the core beliefs holding together the businesses of heart surgery, modern pharmacology, cardiac care departments, and food manufacturing is the idea that cholesterol is bad for you. Cholesterol is, of course, a waxy natural substance contained in high levels in eggs, meats, tropical oils, fish, shrimp, and butter. If you're like most people, you've read for many years that saturated fats are very bad for you, and cholesterol is bad for your arteries and your heart. Greatly simplified, the theory goes that if you eat too much cholesterol, it will lodge in your arteries causing them to harden and make you vulnerable to a heart attack.

One of the reasons why the theory that cholesterol is bad for you has been around for so long and is accepted as dogma, is it's a simple idea that people can easily visualize. I'll get to the history of this dogma soon and tell you how successful this unproven theory has been in selling you manufactured foods, supporting the heart surgery business and keeping the ball rolling for Big Pharma, America's most profitable business.

My own steps along a path that might have led me straight to the modern-day sacrificial altar started innocently enough. I went to a health fair at a local hospital in Santa Barbara and got my blood tested for cholesterol. While I was there, I picked up handouts from cheery hospital volunteers stating simple, logical, and self-evident "truths" about saturated fat and cholesterol. They were easy to read, and like so many others have done, I took their message for granted.

The first hand-out was printed by the American Heart Association and was entitled: *How Can I Lower The Bad Cholesterol in My Blood?* The following bulleted answers were offered:

✓ Eat low fat, low cholesterol, high fiber foods.
✓ Cut down on high-fat foods.
✓ Lose weight if you need to.
✓ Ask your doctor about medicine that can reduce cholesterol (not recommended for all patients.)

Further along in the flyer from the American Heart Association, I read a section entitled: *What About Fats?* It explained that there are three different kinds of fats in the foods we eat:

✓ Saturated fat is the kind that raises cholesterol, so it's not good for you. Avoid animal fats like butter, lard and meat fat, and some plant fats like coconut oil, palm oil and palm kernel oil.
✓ Polyunsaturated fats are found in vegetable oils and fish oils. These tend to lower blood cholesterol.
✓ Monounsaturated fats are found in olive, canola, peanut, sunflower and safflower oils. In a low-fat diet, they may lower blood cholesterol.

Surprisingly enough, most of this dietary message from the American Heart Association and the American Medical Association is inaccurate and isn't good medical or diet advice. This may be the first time you've heard this message, but a number of progressive dietary crusaders have been busy challenging the dietary dogma that cholesterol is bad for you, including Sally Fallon, spokeswoman for the Weston-Price Foundation, Mary G. Enig PhD, a leading authority on nutritional oils, and Uffe Ravnskov, MD, PhD.

What these experts have been saying is that cholesterol is not only good for you, but you're making a big mistake by not eating healthy saturated fats found in butter, lard, meat, raw certified milks and cheeses, and coconut oils. These oils are the best for your body. It's a fact that heart disease was almost completely unknown in this country when people ate large amounts of high quality saturated fats. What's bad for you is consuming hydrogenated polyunsaturated oil, or unstable (rancid) oils made from vegetables.

The heart disease epidemic that occurred from the 1920s to its peak in 1968 has strong correlations to the increase in the use of margarines, polyunsaturated oils, and cheap hydrogenated soybean and cottonseed oils. As butter consumption declined during this time period, the use of polyunsaturated vegetable oils increased over 400%. The consumption of cheap oxidized cholesterols in rancid oil and the use of margarine and hydrogenated soybean oils have been a major factor in the rise in heart disease.

As you will see in the next few chapters, there are other factors involved in heart disease, such as lack of exercise, sugar consumption, and the critical lack of vitamins and minerals in the American diet. You need to know that heart disease is almost unknown in primitive peoples and used to be extremely rare in America. The heart disease epidemic correlates almost exactly with the rise in the use of cheap, usually oxidized and rancid, vegetable oils; sugar, white flour, and canned and processed foods. The rise in consumption of processed and canned foods has also deprived Americans of vitamins and minerals in their diet due to the practice by agri-businesses of strip-mining American soils. Cheap chemical fertilizers made from petroleum and squirted into depleted soils do not create healthy foods that make strong bodies.

Heart Disease, Vitamin Deficiencies, and Saturated Fat

Eating the wrong kind of cholesterol is bad for your heart, but the primary cause of heart disease is more closely correlated with vitamin deficiencies. In Chapters 3 and 4, I'm going to give you specific vitamin formulas to prevent and reverse heart disease. Heart disease is not some mysterious evil disease always waiting to strike you down out of the blue. The majority of heart disease is predictable, preventable and highly avoidable.

Despite the brainwashing you've had all your life by "reputable" medical authorities and commercial interests out to make a buck off you, I'm hoping I can convince you that cholesterol in high quality saturated fats is essential to your diet. Not eating enough of the right kind of fats (coconut oil, butter, olive oil and lard) and eating too much of the wrong kind of fats (oxidized cholesterols, hydrogenated soybean oils, and trans fats) sets you up with a double-whammy for bad health.

What I've found in my research is how hard it is for most people to change their beliefs. Most people behave irrationally when their beliefs are challenged. If you're a typical American, you've been brainwashed for so long that the truth seems strange, indeed.

One of those who has challenged the dominant paradigm is Swedish doctor, Uffe Ravnskov MD, PhD, who actually had his book, *The Cholesterol Myths—Exposing the Fallacy that Saturated Fat and Cholesterol Cause Heart Disease*, burned by book reviewers on Channel 2 in Finland. That's censorship when they burn your book in a highly educated and tolerant country like Finland! Even in Sweden and Finland, the powerful dogmas of American organizations like the American Heart Association, the National Heart, Lung and Blood Institute and the American Medical Association have kept the failed theory that heart disease is correlated with your cholesterol levels from close scientific scrutiny.

When you start digging into the *status quo* idea that the cholesterol you eat in your food is deposited in your arteries and causes heart disease, you find this is a theory that's been disproved in many ways, and it does a poor job of covering the facts. Surprisingly enough, modern medicine and research doesn't really understand the exact mechanism of why heart disease occurs. What is known is that high cholesterol levels are only one of many risk factors for heart disease.

The point is this: High cholesterol levels are a symptom of heart disease—not a cause. Cholesterol is found in arterial blockages, but its role is like what happens in a snow ball fight—the last one caught with the snowball in hand—is the one blamed for the fight.

Here are the facts of life about heart disease: "High cholesterol" is only one of at least nine well-known risk factors that may predict the possibility of heart attacks and strokes. The others are heredity, being male, advancing age, cigarette smoking, high blood pressure, diabetes, obesity, and lack of physical activity. The more risk factors you have, the greater the chance of heart disease and stroke.

Perpetuating the Myth

At this point, we should ask the question: How did the failed hypothesis that saturated fats in your diet harden your arteries and cause heart diseases ever reach such wide acceptance? Probably the most powerful proponent of this theory was the late Ancel Keys, a former director of the Laboratory of Physiological Hygiene at the University of Minnesota. He published a scientific paper in 1953 titled *Atherosclerosis: A problem in newer Public Health* that kicked off the national anti-cholesterol campaign. Due to his work with the Department of Defense in publishing research work, Dr. Keys was an energetic and well known scientist who commanded respect from his colleagues. He's also remembered for his work with the military for inventing K-rations and for popularizing the Mediterranean Diet.

One of the erroneous notions perpetuated by Dr. Keys was that the Mediterranean Diet is a low fat diet. This continues to be repeated by many other diet authors over the years. Keys overlooked the fact that the diet of Greek and Crete islanders contains a lot of salami, yoghurts, lamb meat, and other high fat foods. Due to recent affluence—and their high fat diet—Greek women are now among the fattest women in the world.

Other problems with the Ancel Keys cholesterol hypothesis began to surface even back in the early '60s with the work of researchers, such as Professor George Mann from Vanderbilt University. Professor Mann took a mobile laboratory to Kenya to study the Masai people at around the same time as Dr. Gerald Shaper from Makerere University in Uganda went out to study another tribe, the Samburus.

The diet of both of these tribal peoples consisted of nothing but raw milk, meat and blood. For long periods, the Samburus would consume two gallons of milk daily from Zebu cows, which have far higher butterfat levels than milk from Holstein cows in America. Sometimes, the Samburu would also eat two to four pounds of meat each day. The Masai didn't drink as much milk but would eat meat like Native Americans did in pre-conquest times, and eat four to ten pounds of meat at one sitting.

If the cholesterol theory of diet and heart disease were correct, these Africans should have some of the highest cholesterol levels in the world. What researchers actually found was quite a surprise. Both the Samburus and the Masai had among the lowest levels of cholesterol ever measured anywhere in the world! Their average cholesterol levels were less than half of the levels of most Americans. Lucky for them, they'd never been exposed to such medical quackery as the failed hypothesis that heart disease is caused by cholesterol in your diet. Professor Mann later called the cholesterol theory, "the greatest scientific deception of this century, perhaps of any century."

However, the defenders of this failed theory have a lot of money invested in keeping you believing that cholesterol is bad for you. Pfizer alone sold over $13 billion worth of cholesterol lowering drugs in 2006. They're making billions of dollars in profit and will go to almost any lengths to keep you believing that cholesterol is a menace to your health.

Other factors that led the general public to believe saturated fats and high levels of cholesterol cause heart attacks were major studies, such as the Framingham Heart Study that began in 1948. The Framingham study is still quoted as a reference source for those who believe in the diet/heart/cholesterol hypothesis, despite its authority in disproving the hypothesis.

In the study, 5,000 people were followed and studied every five years. The group was divided into two sections: Those who ate large amounts of animal fat and those who ate very little. Forty years after the start of the Framingham Study, Dr. William Castelli, director of the project, reluctantly admitted, "In Framingham, Massachusetts, the more saturated fat one ate, the more cholesterol one ate, the more calories one ate, the lower the person's serum cholesterol. We found the people who ate the most serum cholesterol and ate the most calories weighed the least and were the most active." Famous heart surgeon Michael De Bakey, quoted from a *New York Times* article by Sandra Blakeslee, dated April 9, 1987, also said about the study: "An analysis of cholesterol values....in 1,700 patients with atherosclerotic disease revealed no definite correlation between serum cholesterol levels and the nature and extent of atherosclerotic disease."

Time has shown it's hard to kill even a theory that's been disproved once the bandwagon has been rolling long enough. As nuclear physicist Max Planck said, "A new scientific truth does not triumph by convincing its opponents and making them see the light. But rather, because its opponents eventually die and a new generation grows up that is familiar with it."

The proponents of what has come to be called the "lipid hypothesis" (saturated fats in the diet cause high cholesterol and result in heart disease) are guilty of many scientific errors, such as confusing statistical association with causation, as well as selective citation. Most of the studies, like much of the current research done by large drug companies, were poorly designed and poorly conducted. Many didn't produce the results researchers were looking for and so are often quoted in misleading ways. It's a sad fact, but most of the scientific research today is sponsored by drug companies looking for validation of new drugs that can be marketed to reap huge profits made from selling statin drugs to reduce your cholesterol levels. Salesmanship has trumped science in America when it comes to selling prescription drugs.

The great saturated fats/cholesterol bandwagon was already rolling in the 1950s, and you can still feel the effects almost 50 years later in the sort of errant nonsense handed out by organizations like the American Heart Association at health fairs at your local hospital. This smokescreen about cholesterol has helped food manufacturers sell you foods full of hydrogenated oils and trans-fats (with a shelf life from here to eternity), margarine, vegetable oils, sugar-laden processed foods, and unhealthy low fat foods. And even worse, they've managed to make you fearful of eating heart healthy foods like butter, organ meats, beef, poultry and coconut oils. The real money in the food business isn't in the agriculture side—it's in the "food" manufacturing business.

It's a shame those Samburu and Masai cattle herders in Africa didn't have any of our white jacketed medical experts to drive out into the bush in a shiny black BMW and warn them of the danger of getting heart disease from eating so much cholesterol. The biggest danger to the African cattle herders' health might be in spraining some ribs by laughing so hard at such an absurd idea!

ABOUT CHOLESTEROL:

Your body produces over three to four times more cholesterol each day than the cholesterol you eat.

Eating animal fat and animal foods containing cholesterol do not raise blood cholesterol levels very much.

People with low cholesterol levels are as likely to die of heart disease as those with high cholesterol.

People with low cholesterol are more likely to die of stroke, suicide, cancer, and accidents—especially when cholesterol has been lowered by using statin drugs.

All studies have shown that cholesterol has little or no correlation to being a risk factor for heart disease in women or men over age 50.

Older women with high cholesterol live longer than older women with low cholesterol.

More than 30 studies with more than 150,000 people have shown those who've had heart attacks haven't eaten more saturated fat or less polyunsaturated oil than other people.

Mother's milk contains higher proportions of cholesterol than any other food. Cholesterol plays an important role in brain and nervous system development in infants and young children. As much as 50 per cent of the calories in mother's milk are saturated fat. In light of this, do you think it makes sense for the American Heart Association to recommend low cholesterol and low fat diets for children? Most commercial baby formulas are low in saturated fats. Even worse, soy formulas are completely lacking in cholesterol.

Cholesterol is a precursor molecule for your body's important hormones. This includes estrogen, testosterone, corticosteroids, and progesterone.

Cholesterol acts as an anti-oxidant and protects against free radical damage associated with toxins and advancing age. As we age, our body makes more cholesterol to protect us from damage from free radical toxins.

If you reduce the amount of cholesterol in your diet, your liver will manufacture more cholesterol.

High levels of cholesterol in the blood may indicate your body needs extra protection from deadly toxins, such as sugar, hydrogenated fats, trans fats, margarine, chemically altered fats, synthetic faux fats, such as Olestra and synthetic faux sugars like Splenda.

Your brain and your nervous system have the highest amounts of cholesterol in your body. Your brain is composed of as much as 70% cholesterol and saturated fat.

ABOUT SATURATED FATS:

Saturated fats make up more than 50% of your cell membranes.

The main fuel for your heart's pumping action is saturated fat. (To be specific—it's *stearic acid* and *palmitic acid*.) The fat around your heart stored as a reserve fuel supply is mostly saturated fat.

Saturated fats protect your liver from toxins, such as alcohol and Tylenol, a known liver toxin.

Some saturated fatty acids, such as short and medium chain fatty acids like coconut oil, protect against infection.

Saturated fats are good for the health of our bones, enhance our immune system, and are needed for the utilization of essential fatty acids.

Do you remember the many research reports starting about thirty years ago saying how dangerous eggs are for your health, because they're high in cholesterol? Then along came more research saying that eggs were also high in lecithin which lowers cholesterol. What was a person supposed to believe? Millions of dollars of industrial, synthetic foods are still being sold that are faux food substitutes for eggs, and many dietary "experts" still advise you to eat only the whites of eggs in omelets. Reality is that eggs are nearly a perfect food. It's hard to find a more inexpensive source of high quality protein than eggs raised from free range chickens (not Industrial Chickens).

Cook eggs in fresh butter, olive or coconut oil and enjoy them. They're good for you! Some of the more interesting information in the good Swedish doctor Uffe Ravnskov's book, *The Cholesterol Myths*, is his table showing what happened to his cholesterol levels when he increased his consumption of eggs. What do you think happened to his blood cholesterol levels when he ate eight eggs daily? The table below, reprinted with permission, shows how it dropped!

Table 3B: *Egg consumption and cholesterol values in one skeptical Swedish doctor.*

DAY	NUMBER OF EGGS CONSUMED	BLOOD CHOLESTEROL (mg/dl)
0	1	278
1	4	278
2	6	278
3	8	266
4	8	264
5	8	264
6	8	257
7	8	274
8	8	246

Two Sides of the Cholesterol Coin

Like a lot of the health information in this book, the story of cholesterol illustrates the dual nature of our modern foods. There's an enormous difference between natural, healthy cholesterol in eggs, raw milk, natural meats, sea foods, and organic poultry, and the damaged, oxidized cholesterols found in powdered milk, powdered eggs, and rancid, oxidized polyunsaturated vegetable oils in thousands of manufactured foods. Also, the oxidized cholesterols (trans fats) found in large quantities in fried foods from your average fast food joint are a major source of ill health in America.

Denmark has taken the global lead in not allowing more than 2% trans fats in any foods. Can this change be done on a large scale? Of course it can. When these regulations passed, the fast food behemoths like Burger King and MacDonald's, with a footprint in Denmark, were quick to comply with strict Danish regulations in order to keep selling their defective foods. New York was the first major city to place restrictions on trans fats (oxidized cholesterols) in restaurants within the city limits. They're on the right path, despite the harsh criticisms by prominent business magazines, such as *Forbes*, which sarcastically reported these proposals as being part of the "Nanny Culture."

I freely admit that much of this chapter isn't original. I've taken information from many sources to tell you what you need to know about cholesterol. However, one discovery of mine that is original is my interpretation of the results found from autopsies done by military investigators on young American and Korean soldiers killed in the Korean War. (This discovery has been mentioned in many different health and diet books from *Fit for Life* to most recently, *The China Study*.) Investigators found extremely high levels of atherosclerosis (hardened arteries) and coronary blockages in the hearts of both Koreans and Americans, reporting that 77.3% had gross evidence of heart disease. At least 1 out of 20 had so much arterial plaque that 90% of an artery was blocked. The average age of the 300 young soldiers autopsied was 22 years of age.

The discovery that both groups of soldiers had such severe hardening of their arteries at so young an age was a tremendous surprise. The accepted explanation has been to blame high levels of saturated fats from high meat and homogenized milk consumption. But the problem with this line of reasoning is that the Korean soldiers typically ate a diet much higher in rice, grains and vegetables than the young American soldiers.

What's been overlooked in this story is the heavy consumption by both Korean and American soldiers of oxidized cholesterols in powdered eggs and powdered milk. What did soldiers in the 1950s eat more of than powdered eggs and powdered milk? I'm sure they also ate a lot of the greasy fried foods in Army chow lines of that era that were also high in damaged cholesterols.

It's a sure bet that both groups (Koreans and Americans) were exposed to large amounts of oxidized cholesterols and their diet was lacking in fresh vegetables, fruits and vitamins. Also, like all combat soldiers, they lived every day with an enormous amount of stress. The message, I believe, from these autopsies is that when people are exposed to large quantities of oxidized cholesterols, high levels of stress, and eating a diet deficient in vitamins and minerals, atherosclerosis can develop quickly, even in young people.

Before I learned what I know about cholesterol, I thought it was useful to drop my cholesterol levels a great deal and to avoid eating saturated animal fats, butter and animal proteins. I realize now that by eating lean seafood, vegetables and tofu and by eating only small amounts of red meat and butter, I was forcing my body to make more cholesterol, because I was depriving it of cholesterol from healthy, natural sources. If you feel it's healthy to have extremely low levels of cholesterol, the best way to lower cholesterol levels is by fasting and using nutritional supplements.

HOW TO HAVE A HEALTHY HEART

Eat ample amounts of healthy cholesterol contained in meats, butter, seafood, organ meats.

Cut back drastically on your sugar intake and consumption of processed foods (white flour, pastas, white rice, crackers, potato chips, etc.). Eating too much processed food prevents you from eating natural foods containing essential vitamins B, C, and E.

Never eat trans fats, skim milk, 1% or 2% milk, hydrogenated oils, corn oils, soy bean oils, margarine, Egg-Beaters, and Crisco. Avoid oxidized cholesterol found in rancid cooking oils, and the ubiquitous powdered eggs and powdered milk in many processed foods.

Cut all tobacco usage, a well documented vector for heart disease.

Heart Disease and Inflammation

Most of the current research on the causes of heart attacks and stroke is now focused not on cholesterol but on three other indicators: inflammation, homocysteine (a sulfur containing amino acid) levels, and C-reactive (CPA) protein levels. I'm talking here about the real research, not the many phony trials and studies funded by large drug companies, to obtain results to justify the sale of more statin drugs to lower "bad" cholesterol for larger segments of the population and to sell new drugs to raise your "good" cholesterol. In the next chapter, I'll give you information about a simple blood test that's a more accurate assessment of your risk of heart disease and stroke than serum cholesterol levels. My homocysteine test cost $85. You should get tested too—it just might save your life.

Among almost all serious researchers, atherosclerosis is now recognized as an inflammatory disease. This model of heart disease helps explain why LDL cholesterol can be a risk factor. In the next chapter, I'm going to explain how LDL cholesterol carries homocysteine acids, and if the levels of LDL are excessively high, they cause hardening of your arteries. Taken from good scientific evidence, the inflammation model of heart disease, hardening of the arteries and occlusive stroke is consistent with the known facts.

According to this model of heart disease, problems start when LDL particles collect in the internal lining of arteries. This is not a problem until these LDL particles become oxidized or change their molecular shape into a form your immune system recognizes as abnormal and triggers an inflammatory response. Newly discovered markers of inflammation, such as C-reactive protein, are currently being used as indicators of heart attack risk. *Testing your homocysteine levels and for C-reactive protein is the best way to access your risk of cardiovascular disease.*

The role of infection in heart disease is now being taken seriously by many researchers and is supported by reports that both bacteria and viruses have been found in arterial plaque tissue. There is even some consideration of treating heart disease with antibiotics. As I mentioned earlier, the overall health of your teeth and your gums is an excellent indicator of the health and condition of your cardiovascular system. (Before you get too concerned about your gingivitis—take at least 2,000 to 3,000 milligrams of vitamin C daily for 30 days and see if that stops your gums from bleeding.)

There are at least three explanations for the connection between gum disease and hardening of the arteries. One is that gingivitis-causing microbes can travel in the bloodstream and cause inflammation of your arteries. The second is that low-level infection of your gums secretes chemicals in your blood stream encouraging the growth of arterial plaques. The third mechanism is that high sugar consumption and low anti-oxidant levels produce both gum and heart disease. The link to sugar and heart disease is very strong.

The Truth About Cholesterol-Lowering Drugs

I realize in writing *The Santa Barbara Diet,* I may be offending medical professionals who believe the Holy Grail of preventing heart disease and hardening of the arteries has been achieved by the development of cholesterol lowering drugs, called *statins*. The real truth about these drugs—Lipitor (the number one selling drug in the world), Zocor, Provichol, and Crestor—is they offer small benefits at an enormous cost, with many side effects and adverse reactions, including the risk of death or cancer.

Statin drugs do slightly lower the rate of coronary heart disease, but the mechanism by which they do so isn't well understood. It doesn't appear to be the result of lowering cholesterol levels. It's quite possible whatever benefits derived from the use of dangerous statin drugs come not from their cholesterol lowering properties but from some efficacy in reducing inflammation, stabilizing arterial plaques and reducing clotting. Many chemical drugs have more than one biological effect—this is probably the case with statin drugs—as a large body of research shows that higher or lower levels of cholesterol have little to do with your mortality from heart disease.

Recently, Big Pharma has lobbied the medical establishment into recommending your total cholesterol be lowered from below 200 down to 160, and your LDL, or "bad" cholesterol, should be less than 80. These levels are impossible to achieve without using drugs, and that's the objective of Big Pharma; they want everyone in the world using their dangerous and incredibly profitable statin drugs.

Once you know the difference between "good" cholesterol and "bad" cholesterol, you should realize that for men over 50, cholesterol levels of 220 and 240 are perfectly natural and healthy. Statin drugs should only be taken by those with very high cholesterol levels (over 300) or those with reduced life expectancy due to heart disease.

The medical industry, food manufacturers, and Big Pharma have a lot at stake in keeping you in the dark on this cholesterol issue. Statin drugs have been the most profitable drugs in American history. There's a lot of money to be made by funding phony studies, bribing doctors, and keeping you confused as to the truth about BIG BAD EVIL CHOLESTEROL. Since advertising for drugs on TV became legal in 1997, they've pulled out the stops on ads to make you think your very life itself depends upon lowering your cholesterol levels. Just to give you an idea of how big the money made in the drug industry is, in 2002, the combined profits of the ten drug companies in the Fortune 500 ($35.9 billion) were more than the profits for the other 490 businesses put together ($33.7 billion).

Ultimately, you must make your own decision whether you are one of the few people, perhaps less than 1%, of the current users of statin drugs, who can benefit from their use. But if you want to take statins, I suggest you try natural statin drugs, such as Chinese red yeast rice that has been used as a health aid in Asia for centuries. Of course, taking red yeast rice is a lot cheaper than Lipitor. Each dose costs less than one tenth of 1% of what a dose of Lipitor costs. And because they're naturally occurring substances, not patented chemicals made to mimic the effects of naturally occurring yeast strains, they have few, if any, side effects. If you do choose to take statins, why not take inexpensive, natural ones?

More Fraud: Statins for Cancer, Stroke Prevention and Heart Failure

Of all the various frauds in this chapter, the attempts to prescribe Lipitor and Zocor to prevent cancer might be the biggest lie of all. Despite the fact there have been studies published since 1996 linking statin drugs to cancer in lab animals, Big Pharma hasn't quit trying to jury-rig randomized studies to get the green light for claiming that statin drugs prevent cancer.

In 1996, a team of researchers from San Francisco University Medical School showed that cholesterol-lowering drugs cause cancer in laboratory animals at amounts that are being prescribed to tens of millions of people. Why did the FDA allow the approval of these dangerous, known carcinogenic drugs? The UCSF researchers answered the question by revealing, "The pharmaceutical companies manufacturing these drugs downplayed the importance of these side effects and thereby removed any obstacles for their approval." Hundreds of millions of dollars are being spent for advertising annually, promoting the use of statin drugs that are known to cause cancer.

So far, none of Big Pharma's research and funding efforts to get cholesterol lowering drugs approved as cancer fighting drugs have delivered any results. A recent article the *Wall St. Journal* reported findings from *Journal of the American Medical Association*: "Contrary to some researcher's hopes, cholesterol-lowering statin drugs do nothing to fight cancer, an analysis found. Researchers analyzed 26 rigorous, randomized studies involving more than 73,000 patients and concluded that drugs such as top selling Lipitor and Zocor had no effect on cancer risk or cancer deaths."

Since attempts to have Lipitor marketed for use in cancer didn't work out, Pfizer, the manufacturer of Lipitor, has been busy funding large studies trying to claim that Lipitor also prevents strokes. Actually, just like the cancer story, the evidence from a recent study showed Lipitor caused almost twice as many hemorrhagic strokes (brain hemorrhages) in patients who took the drug as in those who took a placebo.

Here's a quote from a story printed in the *Wall Street Journal* on August 11, 2006, with a headline reading: *Lipitor Shows Limited Benefit for Stroke:* "A new study sponsored by Pfizer Inc. found the company's best-selling drug, Lipitor, had only modest success in lowering the stroke rate in people with prior strokes, while raising red flags concerning a higher incidence of potentially devastating brain hemorrhages." When you read a little further in the article, you find this line: "But the strokes which occurred in Lipitor patients included 55 hemorrhagic strokes, which can be particularly devastating, compared with 33 such events among patients getting a placebo."

To be fair to Pfizer and Lipitor, I should tell you about the benefits of this trial too: "Among the patients who took Lipitor, 265 patients, or 11.2% of the total Lipitor group, suffered another stroke over five years. That compared with 311 patients, or 13.1%, of those getting placebo pills who suffered additional strokes." Rochelle L. Chaiken, Pfizer's world-wide medical director, is quoted as saying, "The benefit is clearly there," in terms of stroke reduction in people with previous strokes, adding, "We're very excited about the data."

Pfizer's spin on the data is simply staggering. When you look at the positive tone in the headline, also, you realize that Pfizer, Inc. is one of the *Wall St. Journal's* best customers for buying advertising space. How would you like to be one of the 22 people in this test that had a devastating hemorrhagic stroke in your brain courtesy of the Lipitor you used in the test? Obviously, it was a lot safer to take the placebo. Please Pfizer, give me the placebo, or give me death.....

In a side note about Pfizer, the company was recently sued by an employee insurance fund of the State of New Jersey over allegations that Pfizer defrauded state and federal Medicaid programs by marketing Lipitor to broader populations of patients than permitted under federal rules. This lawsuit filed in Federal Court in Newark, New Jersey, alleges that Pfizer illegally sought to persuade doctors to prescribe an expensive, life-long drug regimen to patients with only low to moderate heart disease risk, in violation of its federally approved labeling. The lawsuit states that a 2004 Pfizer securities filing "blatantly promotes Pfizer's off-label use as a business opportunity for Pfizer."

After three years of reading *Forbes, Barron's, Fortune* and the *Wall Street Journal* doing research for this book, it's obvious to me that Pfizer's strategy is *full speed ahead—damn the torpedoes—pay the lawyers—keep doing anything possible to make a buck*. After all, Pfizer reported Lipitor sales of $12.1 billion in 2005. Their total sales since 2001 are over $46 billion.

Pfizer has already done an end run around these minor problems by getting FDA approval to prescribe Lipitor to lower the risk of stroke in Type 2 diabetics who don't yet show any sign of heart disease but might be at risk of developing the disease. The kicker here, of course, is that 40 million Americans are at risk of getting diabetes. Hmmmm, Lipitor for you, Sir?

And then there's the link to heart failure. All statin drugs decrease your body's production of ubiquinone (coenzyme Q10) which can weaken your heart muscle and cause it to fail. Since statins have been widely used, there has been a large increase of the numbers of deaths due to heart failure. In a leading medical journal, cardiologist Peter H. Langsjoen refers to the trend as *statin cardiomyopathy*. He stated:

> *Never before has the medical establishment knowingly created a life threatening nutrient deficiency in millions of otherwise healthy people, only to sit back with arrogance and horrific irresponsibility and see what happens. As I see two or three new statin cardiomyopathies per week in my practice, I cannot help but view my once great profession with a mixture of sorrow and contempt.*

Unfortunately, in 1999, Merck & Co. patented and never used two drugs combining CoQ10 with statins to prevent CoQ10 depletion and diminish other serious side effects.

My question is: *Do you spell fraud with a small "f" or a capital "F?"*

The Doctors Speak

I'm going to end this chapter with a few quotes from doctors who have spoken out against the massive fraud perpetuated every day in the name of lowering your cholesterol levels.

Paul J. Rosch, M.D. is a clinical professor of medicine and psychiatry at New York Medical College, editor of three medical journals and former president of the New York State Society of Internal Medicine. As cited in *Stop Worrying About Cholesterol,* by Richard Tapert, Dr. Rosch wrote:

> *A massive crusade has been conceived to lower your cholesterol count by rigidly restricting dietary fat, coupled with aggressive drug treatment. Much of the impetus for this comes from speculation, rather than any solid scientific proof. The public is so brainwashed that many people believe that the lower your cholesterol, the healthier you will be, or the longer you will live. Nothing could be further from the truth.*
>
> *The cholesterol cartel of drug companies, manufacturers of low fat foods, blood testing devices, and others with huge vested financial interests have waged a highly successful promotional campaign. Their power is so great they have infiltrated medical and government regulatory agencies that would normally protect us from such dogma.*

Edward Pinkney, M.D., editor of four medical journals and former co-editor of the *Journal of the American Medical Association,* wrote in the beginning of his 1973 book, *The Cholesterol Controversy:*

> *Your fear of dying, if you happen to be one of the great many people who suffer from this morbid*

preoccupation, may well have made you a victim of the cholesterol controversy. For if you have come to believe that you can ward off death from heart disease by altering the amount of cholesterol in your blood, whether by diet or drugs, you are following a regimen that has no basis in fact. Rather, you as a consumer have been taken in by certain commercial interests and health groups who are more interested in your money than your life.

CHAPTER THREE

The Homocysteine Revolution

I hope what you've read so far has caused you to start questioning the outdated theories that allow the medical/industrial complex to make gigantic profits by selling you drugs that are not only dangerous, but unproven in their long term effects. What I've learned is *prevention*—not *treatment*—is the future of medicine.

We get so impressed with the incredible technological face of modern medicine, that we forget how medicine, like so many other human endeavors, has been wrong about much during its history. Like all of science, the current best practice tends to dominate the field in medicine, continuing for a long period of time until it is conclusively proven wrong.

The frightening thing is that the best medical practices, even those offered by top doctors and surgeons, can turn out to be totally wrong, given enough time. When I read about former President Bill Clinton's heart attack and heart surgery, I wondered if it couldn't have been prevented by a simple practice, not yet common in the field, of testing *homocysteine* levels in your blood. If Bill Clinton had known he was at risk for heart disease, would he have taken the steps to avoid having a heart attack? Obviously, as a former President of the United States, he had the best medical care possible—yet he still had a heart attack.

Misinformed Treatment

Is it possible the doctors who treated Bill Clinton's heart attack were as misinformed about the cause and treatment of disease as those who treated General George Washington in 1799 when he came down with a cold?

In spite of a storm bringing hail, sleet and snow, George Washington maintained his regular routine and rode his horse for five hours in a storm, then chose not to change his wet clothes when he arrived at

Mount Vernon. Dinner was ready and he didn't want to keep his guests waiting. The next day he had a sore throat, but he still went out in stormy weather and marked trees for cutting. He thought he'd caught a cold, but he said, "Let it go as it came." He felt the best thing to do was simply ignore it.

In the middle of the night, he awakened Martha Washington, and told her his throat hurt and he was having difficulty breathing. At dawn, Martha sent word to fetch Dr. James Craik, George's personal physician and friend of over 40 years. Dr. Craik diagnosed Washington's condition as serious and dispatched riders to bring two local physicians to Mount Vernon to assist.

George Washington received the best possible medical care that science of his era could provide. Unfortunately, every treatment he was given only made matters worse. His physicians bled him four times and extracted more than five pints of blood. They blistered him around his neck and administered powerful laxatives in a misguided attempt to purge his body of infection. If antibiotics had been available then, almost surely, he would have survived.

After studying the evidence, modern medical experts have concluded Washington probably had a bacterial infection of the *epiglottis*, a flexible piece of cartilage at the entry to the larynx. As the epiglottis swells with an infection, it closes off the windpipe and makes swallowing and breathing difficult. The patient has the sensation of being strangled to death by involuntary muscles he can't control. George Washington's last hours must have been painful, as he was being tortured to death by his doctors at the same time. On the evening of December 14th, 1799, George Washington told his doctors to stop treating him and let him go in peace. "Doctor, I die hard—but I am not afraid to go," he said.

Do you think it possible that President Bill Clinton's treatment for his heart attack might cause doctors of the future to look back and shake their heads at how misinformed his treatment was? Would his heart attack have occurred if he had taken the preventative vitamin and mineral formulas for heart disease I'm recommending in this chapter and the next one? That's a question that begs for an answer. The facts of life are such that you can be the President of the United States, receiving the best official medical care, and still be horribly misinformed.

A recent reminder of why you should keep an open mind about

medical treatments is the 2005 award of a joint Nobel Prize for Medicine to two Australian physicians. Drs. Barry J. Marshall and Dr. J. Robin Warren discovered stomach ulcers were not caused by stress or spicy foods. Instead, the culprit is a certain stomach bacterium, *Helicobacter pylori*, which can be treated with antibiotics. Centuries of wrong treatment and misdiagnosis went out the window with their findings. Ulcers had always been believed to be a lifestyle disease caused by too much stress. The treatment had been to take time off from work, chew food more thoroughly, not eat spicy food, eat anti-acids and drink large quantities of milk. Many patients also underwent surgery to have the linings of their stomach removed.

It was way back in 1983 when Dr. Marshall first proposed at a Brussels conference that peptic ulcers might have a bacterial cause. His findings were dismissed by his colleagues as "the most preposterous thing ever heard," according to an entry in *Current Biography Yearbook*. Dr. Marshall persisted with his research and, along with his collaborator Dr. J. Robert Warren, even tested his theory out by using various microbes on his own stomach. Today the milk-and-rest cure is a thing of the past, surgeries are rare (let's hope so), and four million Americans annually are treated with antibiotics to be free of symptoms within weeks. Another question is: *Why did it take 20 years for this to be accepted?*

Back to the heart of our story—I hope some of this information helps you out with your heart—the heart I'm sure you're most concerned about.

Homocysteine Theory: A Dietary Cause of Heart Disease

In 1969, Dr. Kilmer S. McCully first proposed the "homocysteine theory" of heart disease. He stated that when there is too much *homocysteine*, a sulfur containing amino acid, being transported in the blood, arteries become damaged and arterial plaques form. The end result of this process is hardening of the arteries and heart disease. McCully's theory states that one of the primary causes of hardening of your arteries is the lack of adequate amounts of certain vitamins, such as B6, folic acid, and B12 in your diet. Food processing (canning) and refining grains (white flour) destroy both these vitamins.

Dr. McCully proposed the homocysteine theory after learning about a recently discovered disease called *homocystinuria* at a human genetics conference in 1968. This rare disease, which had been discovered in 1962, caused the amino acid homocysteine, usually found only in trace amounts in the blood, to be present in large quantities in the urine of mentally retarded children. In one case, the mother of a nine year old girl diagnosed with homocystinuria told doctors that the girl's uncle had died in the 1930s in childhood of a similar disease. The uncle was severely mentally retarded and had died at age eight of a stroke.

An eight year old dying of a stroke so similar to how elderly people die had been unusual enough for the case to be published in the *New England Journal of Medicine*. The pathologist in this case found the arteries to the young boy's brain were blocked and narrowed by a blood clot that caused the fatal stroke. The pathologist stated the arteries appeared to have the same sort of arteriosclerosis (hardening of the arteries) usually found in elderly patients.

When Dr. McCully researched this early case, he found it had been published by researchers at Massachusetts General Hospital, the same hospital where he was practicing medicine. Because of this coincidental event, he was able to re-examine the original autopsy reports and preserved specimens from the child's organs to confirm the boy had severe arteriosclerosis similar to elderly patients. But the boy's arteries did not have cholesterol or fat deposits in the arterial plaques. Dr. McCully reasoned that the amino acid homocysteine could have produced severe hardening of the arteries and that arteriosclerosis could occur before fats and cholesterol are laid down in damaging plaques in arteries.

A few months later, Dr. McCully learned of another case in which a two month old baby boy who had died of severe pneumonia was diagnosed with homocystinuria. The child hadn't been growing properly, had high levels of homocysteine in his urine, and had a form of the disease apparently caused by an inability to metabolize vitamin B12 and folic acid. Because the earlier case of homocystinuria from the 1930s was caused by an inability to metabolize vitamin B6, the condition of the infant's arteries in this case was crucial. If the child's arteries contained arteriosclerotic plaques, it would prove that homocysteine damages arteries, regardless of which vitamin deficiency caused the elevated levels of homocysteine.

Here are Dr. McCully's own words in re-telling his story: "I barely slept for two weeks. I became very excited because my analysis of these two cases of homocystinuria proved that the amino acid homocysteine was causing arteriosclerosis by directly damaging the cells and tissues of the arteries. Since one case resulted from a lack of vitamin B6 and the other from a deficiency in B12 and folic acid, I could pinpoint the one constant—*a high level of homocysteine in the blood*—as the factor responsible for the arteriosclerosis. If this amino acid produced arteriosclerosis in these patients, then why couldn't homocysteine cause the disease in the rest of the population?"

Dr. McCully also started thinking of other medical experiments that related to these particular cases. Among them were the experiments done on monkeys by the California pathologist James Rinehart in 1949. Rinehart's work had conclusively linked vitamin B6 deficiencies with hardening of the arteries in monkeys. Dr. McCully knew that homocysteine was the missing link that explained the arteriosclerosis. It made sense that a deficiency of B6 caused elevated levels of homocysteine in the blood that caused the monkey's arteries to harden prematurely.

Other studies from Canada involving rats showed that Vitamins B12 and folic acid in their diet also prevented arteriosclerosis. In these studies also, the missing link was homocysteine. If levels in the blood of this sulfur-containing amino acid could be kept low by adequate amounts of vitamins B6, B12, and folic acid in the diet, then hardening of the arteries would not occur.

Dr. McCully's realization that cheap and inexpensive vitamins could be a major factor in preventing and reversing arteriosclerosis was a powerful discovery. It showed that not only in rare cases of homocystinuria and experimental animals, B vitamins were a critical component of healthy arteries and hearts. But as might be expected, Dr. McCully was ostracized for many years by the medical and research community for his theory that homocysteine was a major factor in causing heart disease and arteriosclerosis. Thankfully, a great deal of recent research corroborates and expands upon his theory that homocysteine levels are more important than cholesterol levels in predicting heart disease.

One of the best managed studies that ever attempted to prove high levels of cholesterol cause heart disease was the 14 year long Nurses Health Study. In 1998, investigators from the Harvard School of Public Health published conclusions from this study, showing that 80,000 participants who had the lowest levels of folic acid and vitamin B6 had the highest levels of heart attack and cardiovascular disease. Ironically enough, this study proved that the most critical element in heart disease appeared to be deficiencies of B vitamins, instead of cholesterol levels. These results explain the troubling problem with the cholesterol theory, in that so many cases of heart disease involve patients who don't have elevated cholesterol levels, hypertension, or diabetes.

Check Your Homocysteine Levels

It didn't take much of a leap of the imagination to look at the standard American diet rich in processed foods, white breads, sugar and corn syrup to see that food processing is removing essential vitamins from the foods you eat. When you eat highly processed foods (look around the average American supermarket) you quickly realize most Americans are eating a diet lacking in critical nutrients. If you eat these sorts of foods over long periods of time, the odds are high you have elevated levels of homocysteine that can damage your arteries and your heart.

When I first read Dr. McCully's book, *The Heart Revolution*, I made an appointment with a local doctor, had some blood drawn, and had a homocysteine plasma test done. Being age 55 at the time and male, I quickly realized it was a heart disease prevention test more important than paying attention to my cholesterol levels. The acceptable range of this homocysteine test was listed as 5-12 (micromoles per liter). I was relieved to find my reading was 9.88, well within the acceptable range. The test cost me $85 and is worth doing if you want to assess your risk of heart disease.

However, Dr. McCully stated in his book the optimum homocysteine level was 8. He said that a range between 8-10 was probably safe but should be considered borderline, and one should strive for a lower level. Since I do everything I recommend in this book and have no history of heart disease in my family, I'm not sure that this level isn't too stringent for someone like me.

If your homocysteine level is between 8 and 12, you should make sure you take daily multiple vitamins containing 30 mg. of B6, 100 mcg B12, 400 mcg folic acid. To ensure your heart is healthy, I also suggest you take one tablespoon of brewer's yeast, 400 to 800 I.U. units of natural vitamin E, and at least 2,000 to 3,000 milligrams of vitamin C. You should also change your diet to cut back drastically on sugar, trans fats, and hydrogenated oils. Eat more fresh fruits and vegetables and eliminate processed foods as much as possible.

If your homocysteine level is 15 or higher, you have elevated levels and should consult a physician. The odds are that you are at risk of heart disease and hardened arteries. Your physician should make sure your elevated homocysteine levels aren't being caused by thyroid disease, kidney problems, or diabetes.

Other Factors That Elevate Homocysteine

One thing to keep in mind regarding the homocysteine theory is that factors other then eating a nutrient deficient diet can also elevate your homocysteine levels. These other factors are your genetic background, diabetes, high blood pressure, smoking, aging, and inability to exercise.

Genetic factors may be affecting our high homocysteine levels. Globally, as much as 15% of the population has a genetic defect affecting the ability to metabolize homocysteine. One of the enzymes all of us have, *methylenetetrahydrofolate reductase*, combines with folic acid and lowers homocysteine levels. People born with abnormalities involving this enzyme need to take much higher levels than normal of folic acid to balance out homocysteine levels. Do you have a strong family history of heart disease? Your family history of heart disease might have been caused by this genetic defect, which causes low levels of folic acid in your blood. This is a simple problem which can easily be remedied by taking higher levels of folic acid than others who don't have this genetic defect.

If you have a family history of heart disease, you should get tested with the new homocysteine test which was made available in 1998 for use in clinics and hospitals. If you have a family history of heart disease, you should be supplementing your diet with 50 mg. of B6, 500 mcg B12, and 2,000 mcg. of folic acid.

And finally, the balance of foods that you eat can also elevate your homocysteine levels. *Methionine*, an amino acid that is one of the essential building blocks of protein, is present in large quantities in dairy products and in meats, and in your body, methionine is converted into homocysteine. If your diet is high in meat and dairy products and low in B vitamins, too much methionine is converted into artery damaging homocysteine.

However, if you eat enough foods high in B vitamins, such as organ meats, bananas, lentils, sea foods, fresh meats or whole grain foods, or even take supplements containing adequate folic acid, B6 and B12, then excess homocysteine can be excreted from your body. In other words—if you're going to eat a lot of meat and dairy products, like the average American diet, you need to eat lots of fruits and vegetables, or you need to run 20 miles a day like a Masai cattle herder, to burn it off.

A History of Heart Disease

The good news about heart disease is the rather surprising news of how the rate of heart attacks and death from heart disease has fallen sharply since the late 1960s. You haven't heard much about this because the reasons for the sharp fall in heart disease aren't due to modern medicine's treatments of statin drugs, better surgical techniques, antibiotic-coated stents, or more accuracy in measuring and testing for cholesterol. The rate of heart disease and heart attacks has fallen because of the increased use of vitamin and mineral supplements by the general populace. Another factor in the drop in heart disease is the reduction in the number of smokers.

Let me give you a little history of heart disease: The first diagnosis of a heart attack in medical literature dates back only as far as 1912. Early in the last century, heart disease was extremely rare. There are still many who think that heart disease existed—but simply wasn't diagnosed—as heart disease. This is simply not true.

In the recent book *The China Study*, published in early 2005, author T. Colin Campbell presents statistics to demonstrate how rare heart disease can be in a population that doesn't eat a diet as toxic to the heart as the American diet. In a three year study period between 1973 and 1975, out of 246,000 men in a Guizhou county and of 181,000 women in a Sichuan county, not a single person died of coronary heart disease before age 64! The landmark China Study, probably the largest examination of dietary influence upon disease that will ever be done, also showed the death rate in the early 1970s from coronary heart disease was 17 times higher among American men than rural Chinese men. And for American women, the death rate from breast cancer was five times higher than rural Chinese women.

I thought the *China Study* was a good read compared to most health books—but I reached quite different conclusions than Dr. Campbell does from the data he reported. One of the problems with comparing this data taken from rural peasants in China in the early 1970s with people from affluent Western societies is that Chinese peasants don't necessarily demonstrate the inherent health of the "plant-based diet" and vegetarian regimen that Dr. Campbell advocates in his book. What was really being measured with these statistics was the near starvation of the Chinese peasantry under Mao Tse-Tung's rule.

If you read the story of Mao Tse-Tung in the book *Mao, The Unknown Story* by Jung Chang and Jan Holliday, you'll read that the hungriest years for Chinese peasants were right after the Great Famine of 1958-1961, and the years after Nixon's visit, from 1973 to 1976. To gain influence and attempt to dominate the Communist world, Mao exported sausages and hams to East Germany, funded other tyrants like Mobutu in Zaire, and built expensive infrastructures including railroads and shipyards for countries much more affluent than China. The total Chinese foreign aid expenditures peaked in 1973 at a staggering 6.92 % of GNP. This was over 70 times the level of foreign aid spent by the USA. Meanwhile, almost one billion Chinese peasants lived at near starvation levels.

My point is that the statistics showing how low the rate of heart disease and breast cancer was in China between 1973 and 1975 actually reflected the near starvation of a large rural population. Yet in the book, these statistics were being used to extol the virtues of a plant-based diet.

Not to digress too far, Mao Tse-Tung was a tyrannical ruler who killed more human beings than any other leader in world history. To Mao's credit, during his rule from 1949 to 1976, life expectancy in China increased from 32 years to 65 years, and the literacy rate increased from 15% to 80%. These are solid achievements, especially when compared to how the percentage of Chinese covered by public health programs has plunged from 90 % to only 4%, since capitalism was restored in 1976. However, despite near hysterical adulation for his legacy among many contemporary Chinese, Mao will go down in the history books as a tyrant who ruled over more people for a longer time than anyone in history. His legacy is that of a mass murderer, whose personal choices caused the deaths of more human beings than any leader in world history.

What the China Study from the early '70s actually demonstrates is this: Being close to starvation gives you what modern medicine considers optimum cholesterol and blood pressure levels! If you want to really lower your cholesterol levels and improve your blood pressure, stop eating for a while and they'll fall like a rock. In Chapter Nine of this book, I document a 16 day fast which dropped my own blood pressure levels from 120/90 all the way down to 102/70. My cholesterol levels also dropped precipitously. Only two things have solid scientific evidence of prolonging human life, and they are: anti-oxidants and caloric deprivation, the latter being a clear-cut factor in the study done in China.

But getting back to the history of heart disease in America....

Heart disease was very rare in the 1920s when a young internist named Paul Dudley White introduced electrocardiograph machines from Germany to his colleagues at Harvard University. These machines revealed arterial blockages and allowed early diagnosis of coronary heart disease and hardening of the arteries. In those early days, clogged arteries were such a medical rarity that Dr. White had to search for patients who could benefit from electrocardiography. His colleagues advised him to concentrate on a more profitable branch of medicine, as heart disease was such a rarity.

Later on, during the peak years of heart disease in the '50s and '60s, Dr. Paul Dudley White's name became a household word when he treated President Eisenhower's heart attack. Dr. White's classic textbook, *Heart Disease*, had been published in 1943, and when he began his career, half of all Americans still lived on small family farms and over 80% of the fats they ate were saturated animal fats. People feasted on butter, raw whole milk, eggs and fatty meats, and heart disease was almost unknown.

What changed since the 1920s is the result of a dramatic dietary experiment that no other country has done on such a large scale as America. Some experts estimate that dietary cholesterol intake has only changed about 1% in the last 80 years. Americans are eating relatively comparable levels of cholesterol in their foods, yet we now have much higher levels of heart disease. Why is this? The answer lies in the consumption of dietary vegetable oils, such as margarine, shortening and refined oils, which has increased over 400% in that time period. Also, consumption of sugar and processed foods has increased at least 60% or more.

Modern medical science didn't completely understand how a heart attack occurs until the 1930s, but from the 1930s onward, heart disease became an epidemic that rose sharply until it peaked in 1968. The numbers of heart attacks began to decline in 1968, and are currently less than 50% of levels reached during the late 1960s. Probably the single largest cause of this decline in heart disease has been the use of B Vitamins and other heart beneficial vitamins, such as C, E, and trace minerals, such as selenium and magnesium, by large segments of the population.

In the recent best-selling book *Freakonomics*, authors Steven Levitt and Stephen Dubner examine a sociological trend that is similar to how heart disease has fallen so sharply since the late 1960s. They looked at why crime rates fell sharply in the mid 1980s when all of the experts in criminology expected crime rates to soar. Criminologists had based their expectation on demographic statistics that predicted large numbers of young people would be reaching the age at which most crime occurs. Yet, exactly the opposite occurred.

Crime rates fell precipitously and there were plenty of politicians breaking their arms patting themselves on the back for their great success. Of course, the politicians felt it was their efforts in putting more police on the streets, better tactics for fighting gangs, and expert police work that had reduced crime.

Good statistical analysis by the authors of *Freakonomics* showed the real reason for the drop in crime had been the legalization of abortion. Statistically, children born in families headed by single mothers and without a father in the home have a far higher chance of becoming criminals. It sounds cruel and harsh to speak of so bluntly, but anyone who's studied crime knows that every child being a wanted child, born into a loving and nurturing home, would change the world more than anything else.

You're not alone if you're surprised to hear the incidence of heart disease is less than half of what it was 30 years ago. The National Institute of Health has recently sponsored more than one conference trying to understand the substantial decline in heart disease. Their conclusion was that none of the factors they examined could explain the major statistical decline in heart disease. The facts they had to understand and couldn't went like this: Blood cholesterol levels have declined only slightly (Remember: your diet has little to do with reducing blood cholesterol levels), the total amount of fat eaten has increased only slightly, and other factors, such as more exercise, better medical treatment, and people quitting smoking weren't significant factors in explaining such a drastic decline in heart disease.

The question begs an answer: *Why did heart disease rates fall so sharply since the late 1960s?* One possible explanation is that food processing companies in the late '60s and early '70s started voluntarily adding vitamin B6 to breakfast cereals and to products made from bleached flours. Also, in the 1970s, many more Americans started taking multiple vitamins containing adequate amounts of vitamins C, E, B6, B12, and folic acid. Also, because of better transportation and distribution, fresh produce rich in B vitamins has been available year round. The late 1960s and early 1970s also marked the advent of the natural foods movement in the U.S.A.

Vitamins and Disease Prevention

I realize that many of those in the food processing and medical industries might choose to argue with my conclusions that the primary cause of heart disease in America is vitamin deficiencies. But they should stop for a few minutes and think of the other diseases that have been eliminated by adding vitamins to our diet. Some of the greatest advances in nutritional science in the last century have been the near elimination of the diseases of beriberi, pellagra, rickets, and goiter.

You haven't heard them mentioned recently, have you? That's because all three have been eliminated by adding adequate vitamins and minerals to our modern diet.

Beriberi reached epidemic proportions in India and Indonesia in the early 1900s, when processed white rice, the "new food of civilization," was introduced. When the processing of healthy brown rice into modern white rice began, large numbers of people in Indonesia and India lost the most important source of vitamin B1 in their diet and consequently developed beriberi. White rice is now fortified with vitamin B1.

Pellagra was common in the early 1900s when many people in the southern U.S. lived on grits made from white corn hominy, lacking in niacin (vitamin B3). All processed corn products are now fortified with niacin, and pellagra is a disease of the past.

Rickets is a disease that used to cause bone deformities in children, but with the addition of synthetic vitamin D to milk, it has been almost totally eliminated. Of course, if you drink certified raw milk—with large quantities of healthy natural vitamin D—you won't need to have synthetic vitamins made from petroleum by-products added to your milk. Only adulterated, fractionated, pasteurized, homogenized milk needs to have vitamins added to prevent you from getting diseases.

Goiter is another disease caused by insufficient iodine in the diet and has also been almost totally eliminated by adding iodine to table salt. In a later chapter, I'll give you the scoop on why you should avoid eating common table salt—or "industrial salt"—as I call it. Real Salt is a natural product that's good for you and a boon to your health.

Despite the homocysteine theory being proposed and tested in population studies over the last 25 years, the medical establishment still refuses to acknowledge the link between heart disease and vitamin deficiencies. Don't hold your breath waiting for the FDA to approve fortification of foods with folic acid or B6, either. The only significant change that has been made in recent years is that the Required Daily Amount (RDA) of folic acid has been re-instated at 400 micrograms daily. Also, cereals have been fortified with 140 micrograms per 100 grams, which is a small, but significant amount of folic acid.

This change wasn't done to help protect you and your family against heart disease, but rather because over 25 years ago, it was discovered that adequate levels of folic acid in the diet almost eliminates neural tube defects (*spina bifida*) in newborn babies. Medical studies done during the 1990s proved this connection beyond any doubt. The fortification of cereals and bread has been a major factor in reducing neural tube defects. Some of the reduction in heart disease has been an incidental side effect of a vitamin fortification policy undertaken for a different reason.

Heart Disease Prevention Recap

To summarize what I've said about heart disease, the primary cause of heart disease is a bad diet with low levels of anti-oxidants, high levels of oxidized cholesterols, and a critical lack of vitamins C, B6, B12, vitamin E, folic acid and magnesium. Also, being physically inactive is bad for your heart, and sugar and tobacco usage is also bad news for your heart.

Unless your cholesterol levels are extremely high, you can forget about your cholesterol level being much of a factor for heart disease. To find out your risk of heart disease, I can't urge you enough to get tested for your homocysteine level. This is critical, and you also need to test your level of inflammation by measuring your levels of C-reactive protein (CRP). The C-reactive protein test measures you for molecules produced by the liver in response to inflammatory signals. Both of these are good tests that are much more predictive for your risk of heart disease than testing for cholesterol levels.

By this time, I hope you realize that the failed theory that heart disease is caused by dietary cholesterol is just so much nonsense. Actually, it's worse than nonsense—it's one of the biggest frauds in the history of medicine. Heart disease is an inflammatory disease and modern research is showing that inflammation anywhere in your body is a good marker for heart disease.

Just like in horses and livestock, your mouth is an excellent indicator of your overall health. Current evidence suggests that cavities, gingivitis, and missing teeth are better indicators of heart disease than cholesterol levels or triglycerides. The knee jerk advice of many medical writers and health authorities to deal with oral inflammation is to brush your teeth twice daily and floss at least once.

Of course, you should keep your teeth clean, but you'll find you'll have better oral hygiene if you take 2,000 to 5,000 milligrams daily of vitamin C. Within a few months, this will clear up many dental problems. Having bleeding gums is also a symptom of early onset scurvy, which has many links and similarities to cardiovascular disease. Take vitamin C to your limits of bowel tolerance until your bleeding gums heal. Before the advent of processed foods containing sugar, white flour and hydrogenated oils, primitive people all over the world had beautiful, healthy teeth and never brushed or flossed their teeth. The dental hygiene of modern peoples is a poor substitute for an excellent diet of healthy foods full of essential nutrients.

Your Amazing, Natural Heart

Your heart is an amazing organ and you need to do all you can to support its miraculous functions. Every hour your heart pumps 75 gallons of blood. In a day, it pumps 1,800 gallons of blood that keeps your cells nourished with oxygen. And these figures are for when your heart is resting—blood flows can increase as much as 6 times when exercising vigorously. And the individual cells in your body that receive this oxygen have a complexity you can barely imagine. Each cell contains over 20,000 different types of protein and of these; as many as 2,000 types are each represented by at least 50,000 molecules. There are at least 100 million protein molecules in each cell. It's hard to imagine the teeming, immensity of the biochemical universe going on inside us at a cellular level.

Like myself, you might have been exposed recently to the TV ads showing a lean and wiry looking guy, Dr. Robert Jarvik, "inventor of the artificial heart," walking around in a white coat, holding a clipboard and extolling the virtues of the cholesterol lowering statin drug, Lipitor. In another ad, he's in his cosmic mode, rowing a single scull on a misty morning on a beautiful lake; he looks dynamic and intelligent…. *Go Lipitor! Go Lipitor!* How much do you think they paid him to rep the world's best selling drug?

It was a slick ad, but don't forget—when they sell you the sizzle— you're left with the puddle of grease surrounding the flaming, burnt steak.

Reality is, of course, quite different than the dynamic illusions offered you by the "inventor of the artificial heart." No thanks, Robert. I'll take of the heart I already have and pass on the artificial heart.

Recently, journalist Robert Bazell wrote an article mentioning Jarvik and the somewhat questionable medical credentials of Lipitor's spokesman, "Dr. Robert Jarvik, inventor of the artificial heart." Jarvik attended Syracuse University but didn't have good enough grades to get into medical school, so he enrolled at the University of Bologna in Italy but left after two years. He eventually got a master's degree in medical engineering from New York University. After that he went to work for Dr. Willem Kolff, a Dutch physician and inventor who produced the first dialysis machine and worked at the University of Utah. Kolff became Jarvik's mentor and helped him get a medical degree from the University of Utah in 1976, although *Jarvik never practiced medicine or took an internship.* Dr. Jarvik eventually got a patent on a mechanical heart pump named the Jarvik 7, which was the first of his devices implanted into a human. With the help and promotion of the University of Utah and their huge publicity blitz, the first attempt to put the Jarvik 7 into a human caused enormous worldwide interest.

You might remember the story of the dentist Barney Clark who lived with the Jarvik 7, with many complications, for a total of 112 days before he passed on? During TV press conferences and media events, Dr. Jarvik appeared, (strangely dressed in surgical scrubs) along with head surgeon Dr. William DeVries, to brief the world on Barney Clark's condition. The longest any patient lived on the Jarvik 7 was William Shroeder who also had a series of debilitating strokes and died 620 painful days after the surgery. In May of 1988, a *New York Times* editorial called the artificial heart experiments "The Dracula of Modern Technology." The article said, "The crude machines, with their noisy pumps, simply wore out the human body and spirit."

I'm quite sure the artificial heart doesn't work as well as your own beautiful and immaculate heart. They've invented an artificial kidney machine too, but it's the size of a refrigerator, yet a poor substitute that only performs a few of the functions of a natural kidney. They also have artificial heart valves too, but they only last a few years and each time they open and close, they crush some red blood cells. Your heart's valves open and close two and a half billion times over a lifetime and work perfectly each time.

And Now, How to Avoid Heart Disease

Here's what you need to do to avoid heart disease:

Eat less than 50 pounds of sugar annually.

Eliminate trans-fats and hydrogenated oils from your diet.

Never eat margarine or polyunsaturated vegetable oils.

Make sure you eat healthy saturated fats such as butter, lard, beef tallow, coconut oil and palm oil. The healthiest coconut milk, coconut cream and raw coconut available are frozen products from the Philippines. Ask for them at your favorite Asian market. They're better for you than canned coconut milk. As always, fresh is even better for you.

Make sure you take 250 to 500 mg. of magnesium daily. Over 80% of all Americans are magnesium deficient—and it's critical for your heart's functions. If you have kidney disease, check with your doctor and be careful taking magnesium.

Take at least 2,000 to 3,000 milligrams of vitamin C daily. Taking more up to the limits of your bowel tolerance is suggested. This is the minimum that will keep most people from having heart disease.

Take 400 to 800 IU units of vitamin E made from natural sources daily. Only take natural vitamin E, which is labeled d-alpha-tocopherol. *Vitamin E that's labeled dl-alpha-tocopherol is made from petroleum and is useless.* My guess is that over 90% of all vitamin E being sold is the wrong kind and is biologically useless. It's probably even bad for you to take it. Check your bottles and throw away synthetic vitamin E's.

Make sure you take at least at least 30 mg B6, 100 mcg B12, and 400 mcg of folic acid daily.

Take 1 teaspoon of cod liver oil daily. I recommend the lemon flavored Carlson's variety. No fishy taste.

A Natural Prescription for Heart Health

I've hope I've educated you enough to cause you to you take adequate amounts of B vitamins to control homocysteine levels in your blood. Obviously, getting natural vitamins from eating healthy, unprocessed fruits and vegetables raised in rich, organic soils is the best thing you can do for your health. The best way to get large amounts of B vitamins is to eat bananas, beans, lentils, seafood, whole grains, fresh meats, and especially organ meats, such as liver. Take B vitamins to supplement your food and make sure you're protecting your arteries and your heart with essential nutrients.

Think of taking the following amounts of B vitamins as an insurance policy for the health of your heart. Here are my recommendations:

SUGGESTED SUPPLEMENTS TO MANAGE HOMOCYSTEINE LEVELS			
Disease Risk	Characteristics	Plasma Homocysteine	Supplements (Micromoles per liter)
Low	Eating healthy foods.	4-8	No Supplements
Mild	Poor Diet, Over 60	8-12	30 mg B6 100 mcg B12 400 mcg folic acid
Moderate	Poor diet, obese, Smoker, over 60	10-14	10 mg B6 100 mcg B12 1,000 mcg folic acid
High	Family History: Obesity, smoker, Hypertension, high LDL, low HDL	12-20	50 mg. B6 500 mcg B12 2,000 mcg folic acid
Very High	Angina, diabetes, kidney failure, ischemic attacks	16-30	100 mg. B6 1,000 mcg B12 5,000 mcg folic acid

For the sake of your health—avoid canned foods, highly processed grains, corn syrup and sugar. You lose vitamins by eating refined foods that have natural nutrients and vitamins processed out of them. Foods such as white flour, pasta, white rice, crackers, potato chips, etc. have lost as much as 70 to 90% of vital nutrients. Also, canning vegetables removes between 45 to 88% of all trace minerals and vitamins.

Frozen or fresh vegetables are what your body needs. Eating organic foods grown in rich soils fertilized with natural compost will help add vitamins and minerals to your diet. Remember: *Fresh is best.*

As I mentioned earlier, other vitamins and minerals are also important for the health of your heart. Make sure you take adequate vitamin C, vitamin E, and adequate magnesium to drastically cut your risk of heart disease.

CHAPTER FOUR

Vitamin C: The Missing Link To Good Health

As I continued doing my research for *The Santa Barbara Diet*, a number of fortuitous events occurred that helped me develop a new paradigm of how to view the global epidemic of heart disease and avoid being a victim of it. After I found out how dangerous it is to consume oxidized cholesterols, hydrogenated oils, and sugar, and how the lack of B vitamins causes heart disease and hardening of the arteries, I stumbled onto a missing link in understanding the cause of heart disease: low levels of vitamin C in human blood.

No one was more surprised than me when a 64 year old co-worker of mine from Montecito (an affluent community adjacent to Santa Barbara) suddenly checked into our local Cottage Hospital and had a triple by-pass heart operation. In the same surgery, he had one of his heart valves replaced with a valve from a cow's heart. I was surprised because my co-worker appeared to be in good physical shape, and when he was younger, he'd been fit enough to win two gold medals swimming for the USA in the 1960 Olympics.

By this point in my research, I had learned that heart disease was almost completely unknown in America as recently as 75 years ago. But I hadn't yet gotten an answer to the question: *What had changed so much in 75 years that a man fit enough to win gold medals would have major heart surgery by age 64?*

Vitamin C and Prevention of Heart Disease

As I continued piecing the puzzle together, I learned how vitamin C plays an important role in preventing and even reversing heart disease—still another bit of information the pharmaceutical industry doesn't want you to know about. My discovery began while testing recipes with some friends in Santa Barbara and making a mess of their kitchen. I have to confess that at that time, like most of you, I believed the gospel of medical experts and thought that eliminating fat from my diet was the key to good health.

I was busily trying to develop recipes to find more palatable ways of eating tofu and soy products, when my friend Bob told me about a co-worker, a woman named Barbara Kerr, who'd recently gone to the emergency room with symptoms of what appeared to be a heart attack. Barbara's "heart attack" turned out to have a surprising outcome—very different than what one would expect, since she was in her mid-sixties, moderately physically active, and overweight.

Curious, and sensing a missing piece was at hand, I went to the University of California campus in Santa Barbara to interview Barbara Kerr. She told me what had happened: She'd received a call from her husband telling her their dog, a loyal pet for 16 years, was dying. Frantic, she rushed the five miles to her home and arrived just as the beloved pet died. When she tried to revive the animal, she felt as if a sledgehammer had hit her in the chest. Barbara lay down on the floor clutching her breast and gasping for breath, barely conscious as her husband called 911. When the paramedics arrived, they rushed her as quickly as possible to Santa Barbara Cottage Hospital where a team started prepping her for by-pass surgery.

They were giving her an angiogram when the doctor said, "My God, that's remarkable!" She asked, "What's the matter?" Then the surgeon said, "Everything's fine Barbara, you're going home in a few days. There's nothing wrong with your heart. Your heart and blood vessels are pristine—a 16 year old would be lucky to have a heart in such good condition!"

Barbara recovered fully and did not suffer lasting damage to her heart. The "attack" turned out to have been precipitated by emotional stress as a result of the dog's sudden and unexpected death, a diagnosis known as "stress cardiomyopathy." When this happens for some people, their heart is stunned by a massive release of adrenaline, leaving it temporarily unable to contract normally. Patients typically have no coronary disease, but death is probable without any immediate medical intervention. The condition is similar to "fight or flight," but much more adrenaline is released. New research on the condition, nicknamed, "broken heart syndrome" by doctors, suggests there may be some truth to the old idea that a person can be scared to death or die from sorrow, like a character in a romantic novel who dies of a broken heart.

Barbara, who was retiring from her job as a research associate in charge of the Advanced Molecular Biology Lab, appreciated my interest in the story of her "heart problem" and was most helpful in answering my questions. She explained how the doctor in the emergency room had asked her three questions:

Have you ever smoked?

Do you take vitamins?

What kind of exercise do you do?

Surprisingly enough, her only exercise was walking her dogs about two miles on the beach three or four times each week. When she was much younger, Barbara had a riding injury that impaired her capability to exercise strenuously, and she felt she was 50 pounds heavier than she'd like to be. She had never been a smoker and when asked about her dietary habits, she said she liked to cook her steaks in butter! She drank whole milk, ate organic foods, and the most notable thing about her dietary practices was that she had been taking a full spectrum of vitamins for almost 40 years. The most interesting thing she currently did was taking 800 I.U. units of vitamin E and 10,000 to 15,000 milligrams of vitamin C daily. She took the buffered variety of vitamin C (sodium ascorbate) available from Bronson Laboratories.

When I asked her how and why she had decided to take such large doses of vitamin C, she talked about working at the University with Dr. Crellin Pauling, Ph.D., a genetics researcher and the son of Linus and Alva Pauling. Barbara also had the good fortune of meeting Crellin's father, the genius scientist and humanitarian, Linus Pauling. In talking about him, Barbara told me, "He was one of God's gifts to us."

The Linus Pauling Legacy

I was young and very healthy in the early 1970s and hadn't paid much attention to how Linus Pauling was maligned in the popular press after the publication of his book, *Vitamin C and the Common Cold*. In hindsight, I realize those attacks have a lot in common with how the popular press has treated the issue of global warming.

If you've seen the Al Gore movie, *An Inconvenient Truth,* you'll be interested to know that of 928 peer reviewed scientific articles published in the last ten years, not a single article states global warming is *not* occurring. The score of scientific articles is 928 *pro* and 0 *con* in the debate over whether global warming is real. Yet, in the popular media in the last 14 years, only 53% of the articles in the mass media stated global warming was a fact or was occurring—and the others contested the idea. So much for the way the "truth" is reported in the mass media!

After listening to Barbara Kerr's story about vitamin C, I went down to my favorite used bookstore and was lucky enough to find a signed copy of Linus Pauling's last health book *How to Live Longer and Feel Better,* published in 1986. By reading his own words, one gets a different picture of the consummate scientist, the legendary Dr. Pauling, than you might have received from the mass media spin. It's hard to reconcile the media story of an aging scientist, famous long ago as a nuclear physicist and chemist, overstepping the bounds of his professional discipline and meddling in the field of modern medicine, with the reality of Linus Pauling's life.

Shortly before Linus Pauling died at the age of 93 in 1994, he received a patent for a new technique of fabricating superconductive materials. He also continued his lifelong quest for a peaceful world by speaking out against the first Gulf War in Kuwait. Pauling will be long remembered as one of the giants of modern science and is widely regarded with his friend Albert Einstein as being one of the two most important scientists of the 20th century.

And what a century for science the 20th century was! Rockets to the moon, atomic bombs, computers, the internet, and last, but not least—a cure for heart disease based upon inexpensive vitamin therapies, so that 12 million people don't have to die annually from this epidemic of affluent malnutrition.

The scientific discoveries of Linus Pauling were some of the high points in a long journey that started in a small town in Oregon in the early years of the last century. His career as a chemist began with high school chemistry classes and early experiments he did with "borrowed" materials from an abandoned steel mill near where his grandfather worked as a night watchman. Ironically, he started his brilliant academic career by failing to qualify for a high school diploma, because he didn't take required American history courses. Forty-five years later, after the unprecedented event of winning two Nobel Prizes, his high school was more than happy to award him an honorary diploma.

Pauling did his graduate studies at Cal Tech in Pasadena where his studies of quantum mechanics and quantum theory led him to apply the developing theories to his chosen field of the electronic structure of atoms and molecules. In the 1930s, he began publishing papers on chemistry that led to his landmark textbook, *The Nature of the Chemical Bond*, published in 1939.

In 1941, at age 40, Pauling was diagnosed with a deadly form of Bright's disease, a fatal kidney disease. At that time, most medical experts believed the disease was untreatable. With the help of Dr. Thomas Addis at Stanford University, Pauling was able to control the disease with a low-protein, salt free diet. Unusual for that era, Dr. Addis prescribed vitamins and minerals for all his patients.

During World War II, Dr. Pauling turned over the resources of his laboratories to aid the United States military. He developed missile propellants and explosives for the U.S. Navy and developed an oxygen meter widely used in both submarines and airplanes. President Truman awarded him the Presidential Medal of Merit in 1948 for his endeavors on behalf of the United States during WWII. The irony is that Pauling had been apolitical until WWII, and the experience of WWII caused him to become an international activist for peace until his death.

However, during the McCarthy era, Linus Pauling had his passport revoked and was investigated by the government for his opposition to open air nuclear testing and the military/industrial complex. He was ordered to testify before the Senate Internal Security Subcommittee which labeled him, "the number one scientific name in virtually every major activity of the Communist peace offensive in this country." Under repeated questioning as to the sources of his information, Linus Pauling stated, "Nobody tells me what to think—except for Mrs. Pauling." In the same era, Linus Pauling was once grilled by an FBI agent about how he knew precisely how much plutonium was in a nuclear warhead. His answer was, "I figured it out."

Another of Linus Pauling's accomplishments in the 1940s was his discovery of the cause of sickle cell anemia. In 1945, a friend had discussed the disease with Pauling, and Pauling had used his chemistry training to deduce the disease might be caused by a defect in red blood cell, *hemoglobin*. In 1949, he and his colleague Dr. Harvey Itano published a paper confirming sickle cell anemia was caused by genetic abnormalities in hemoglobin molecules. Pauling called it a "molecular disease," a discovery that laid the foundation for human genome research.

In the late 1950s, Pauling became concerned with the growing problem of air pollution in the Los Angeles area. At that time, most scientists believed smog was caused by chemical plants and refineries— not internal combustion engines. Pauling worked with Arie Haagen-Smit and other scientists at Cal Tech to prove that smog was caused by automobiles. Shortly afterward, Pauling began to work with engineers at the Eureka Williams Company to develop the *Henney Kilowatt*, the first speed controlled electric car. However, Pauling realized early on that traditional lead-acid batteries didn't have enough range or speed to make electrical cars practical or affordable. Pauling recommended that production plans be shelved until the battery problem could be solved, yet the manufacturer pushed ahead. The resulting poor sales were a serious setback for the production of electric vehicles.

Another aspect of the Pauling legacy that has been largely forgotten is his early exposure of the dangers of cigarette smoking. He was one of the first scientists who spoke out against Big Tobacco and cited how dangerous cigarettes are to your health. In the late 1950s, Pauling calculated each cigarette you smoke reduces your life expectancy by about 15 minutes.

In 1958, Pauling and his wife Alva presented the United Nations with a petition signed by over 11,000 scientists, warning the public about the dangers of radioactive fall-out from open air nuclear weapons tests and calling for an end to testing. He also published his book, *No More War*, in 1958.

In 1962, when invited to a dinner at the White House with President John F. Kennedy and his wife Jackie, he spent the day on the sidewalk in front of the White House carrying a placard saying, *Mr. Kennedy/ Mr. McMillan: We Have No Right to Test* protesting against open air nuclear testing. That evening while having dinner with Mr. and Mrs. Kennedy, John Kennedy told Pauling an anecdote of what happened earlier in the day, "When Caroline saw you out there, she asked, 'What has Daddy done wrong now?'" Later in the evening when some lively music was playing after the dinner, Linus Pauling and his wife Alva got up and danced.

I often think what a tragedy it was John Kennedy died in a hail of bullets on that fateful, evil day in Dallas on November 22, 1963. The sixties might have turned out differently if our nation had gone down a different path. After all, JFK had been prescient enough to ask the U.S. Ambassador, while touring Vietnam as a congressman in the 1950s: "What makes you think the Vietnamese will be willing to fight to help keep Vietnam part of France?"

On the same day in 1963 that the Partial Test Ban Treaty was signed by John F. Kennedy and Nikita Khrushchev, Linus Pauling was awarded the Nobel Prize for Peace. The committee described him as "Linus Carl Pauling who, ever since 1946, has campaigned ceaselessly, not only against nuclear weapons tests, not only against the spread of these armaments, not only against their very use, but against all warfare as a means of solving international conflicts."

Linus Pauling's interest in vitamin C began when he met biochemist Irwin Stone, who had attended a lecture by Pauling in New York City in 1966. In the course of the lecture, Linus Pauling stated he was 65 years old, and he hoped to live for another 15 years. Given that both of his parents had died at an early age, and he himself had survived Bright's disease 25 years earlier, he probably had the longevity expectations of an average American in 1966. After the lecture, Pauling visited with Irwin Stone and Stone told him he could live another 50 years if he took large doses of vitamin C.

Irwin Stone had been researching the healing properties of vitamin C since the early 1930s. Both he and his wife had survived serous injuries from a head on car crash with a drunk driver by using large doses of vitamin C, and they felt it had aided the healing process remarkably.

Pauling began a scientific correspondence with Irwin Stone, and he and Alva quietly began taking 3,000 milligrams of vitamin C daily for the next three years. He immediately felt a sense of well being and noticed the colds he'd been plagued with for the last 40 years had almost disappeared.

At first he was skeptical of Stone's ideas, but Stone's theory regarding genetic mutations and vitamin deficiencies intrigued him. Pauling also was aware of George Beadle's research, showing that genetic mutations occurred in mold spores and resulted in the mutated spores having an altered need for nutrients, such as amino acids and vitamins.

Stone had also researched the ability of certain animals to synthesize their own vitamin C in their liver or kidneys. He found that humans, chimpanzees, fruit eating bats, a few tropical birds and guinea pigs were the only mammals lacking the enzyme necessary to synthesize vitamin C. Stone was the first to theorize that the loss of this ability in humans was probably due to a genetic mutation occurring between 25 and 40 million years ago in primates who were the ancestors of modern humans.

The Facts About Vitamin C

The facts about vitamin C are simple: Your body cannot produce a single molecule of vitamin C and without an adequate supply in your diet, you will get scurvy. The adequate amount to avoid scurvy is between 10 and 60 milligrams of vitamin C. If you don't get this amount in your diet, you will die of scurvy. Despite it being known by Portuguese mariners as early as the 1400s that the juice from oranges and limes would heal scurvy, it wasn't until 1911 that scurvy was diagnosed as a vitamin deficiency. Vitamin C (ascorbic acid) was first identified in 1928 by Albert Szent-Gyorgyi who won a Nobel Prize for his discovery.

Vitamin C is a vitamin that's a paradox—you cannot get enough in your diet for optimum protection against heart disease and hardening of your arteries. Adequate supplies of almost all other vitamins can be obtained in your diet—if you eat a diet of the right foods grown in rich, fertile, organic soil. As noted by Linus Pauling, the only way you could get optimum amounts of vitamin C would be to live almost exclusively on a diet of sweet or hot peppers and currants. The fact that almost all creatures have the ability to produce ascorbic acid by their own metabolic processes possibly explains why the supply of this vitamin available through foods doesn't come close to providing optimum amounts.

Linus Pauling recommended that L-ascorbic acid be used as a dietary supplement. Ascorbic acid is a water soluble, crystalline powder that's a synthetic form of vitamin C identical to natural vitamin C from plants. Ascorbic acid is a weak acid only slightly stronger than the acetic acid in vinegar and not as strong as the citric acid in lemons and grapefruit. Almost all of the world's supply is currently manufactured in China from dextrose.

I usually buy ascorbic acid at Trader Joe's for $9.99 per pound. Another good source of vitamin C in quantity is Bronson Pharmaceutical, whose products were used and recommended by Linus Pauling. www. bronsonlabs.com. I like to take their buffered variety of sodium ascorbate as a change of pace from the usual ascorbic acid version. The least expensive way to purchase vitamin C is buying it by the pound.

In addition to the standard ascorbic acid, vitamin C may also be taken as a salt of ascorbic acid, such as *calcium ascorbate* and *sodium ascorbate*. Only these latter two may be taken by injection, if larger quantities need to be taken because of serious illness, such as cancer, HIV, or other life threatening diseases.

A Multitude of Benefits

Research shows that vitamin C (sodium ascorbate) can help fight cancer when taken with intravenous injections, and has powerful, synergistic anti-cancer properties when combined with vitamin K and r-Lipoic Acid. When these vitamins are combined, they enhance the anti-cancer properties of the sodium ascorbate. With such low toxicity and low cost—what better cost/benefit ratio could one hope for in a cancer treatment? There's little to lose—and potentially, a human life to be saved—with this addition to the treatments your doctor prescribes.

If your levels of ascorbic acid are adequate to optimum, it will be present in various body fluids and organs, and especially in the leukocytes and blood. The concentration is also quite high in your brain. Vitamin C's importance for the health of your eyes is strongly indicated because its concentration in the aqueous humor of your eye is very high, almost 25 times higher than blood plasma concentrations.

Vitamin C is absolutely essential in synthesizing collagen, which is a protein that literally holds your body together. Collagen is a white fibrous material, stronger than steel by weight, that forms into networks of elastin making the connective tissue that welds your body together. A person dying of scurvy stops making collagen and literally falls apart—their teeth fall out, their blood vessels break open, their joints fail because their cartilage and tendons deteriorate, and their immune system fails—and then they die.

I wish I'd discovered the good news about vitamin C much earlier than I did. In 2003, I had surgery at age 52 to fuse joints in my toes because I'd worn out the cartilage in them. It took almost four months on crutches and a cane before they healed enough to take the casts off. How I wish I'd known about the doses of vitamin C I should have been taking to heal myself from a surgery like this! These joints never completely healed until almost a year later when I started taking optimum doses of vitamin C. Within a month, the joints had healed better than they did after the surgery. My question then was: *How come physicians and surgeons don't know about this?*

Another benefit of taking substantial amounts of vitamin C is the health of your gums. If your gums bleed when you floss or brush your teeth, you should pay close attention, because recent research shows the health of your gums is closely related to the health of your heart and cardiovascular system. I had gingivitis, an early form of periodontal disease for at least the last five years, despite having regular teeth cleanings and flossing and brushing my teeth twice daily. I was shocked to hear Linus Pauling mention in *How to Live Longer and Feel Better* written in 1986, about the benefits of vitamin C for the health of your gums. To have excellent oral health you need to be taking at least 2,000 to 3,000 milligrams daily.

As Linus Pauling mentioned, the way to avoid getting colds is to take optimum amounts of vitamin C and then, if you feel the small tickle in the back of your throat or any other sign of an impending cold, immediately start taking 1,000 milligrams every hour. Another extremely good health aid for avoiding colds is to take between a teaspoon and a tablespoon of natural brewer's yeast every day. Perhaps there's a synergistic effect with vitamin C and the B vitamins. I mix my vitamin C and brewer's yeast into a small serving of orange or carrot juice.

You should bear in mind that most cold medicines sold over the counter are a toxic witch's brew of nasty chemicals, and should be avoided as much as possible. Billions of dollars are spent every year on medicines that don't prevent colds, but are only palliatives that suppress your cold symptoms and can cause severe side effects.

Vitamin C Dosage

The USDA recommended daily amount is only 60 milligrams which is the amount calculated to keep most people from getting scurvy. Vitamin C is also one of nature's most powerful anti-oxidants and good research has shown that only two things have been scientifically proven to extend human life: caloric deprivation and antioxidants. Why would you want to take less than optimum amounts of a powerful anti-oxidant like vitamin C?

As you're going to see, there's a great difference between the minimum amount needed to prevent you from getting scurvy and the quantity needed for optimum nutrition.

The amount of vitamin C manufactured in the bodies of laboratory rats is estimated to be the equivalent to a 154 pound person taking 1,800 to 4,100 milligrams daily. Yet other animals, such as goats, cows, sheep, mouse, rabbits, cats, and dogs manufacture ascorbic acid at a much higher rate, typically around 10,000 milligrams daily for a body weight of 154 pounds.

Linus Pauling concluded from his studies the optimum daily intake of ascorbic acid for humans should be in the range of 2,300 milligrams to 10,000 milligrams. He also felt there was such wide biochemical variability among different humans, the range might be as great as between 250 milligrams and 20,000 milligrams daily. Good research also shows many common lab animals, such as guinea pigs, manufacture much larger amounts of ascorbic acid when under stress or recovering from injuries.

The amount of vitamin C you should take is best determined by taking it to the limits of your bowel tolerance. It's best to split your daily dose into two or even three portions to make sure you have optimum levels in your blood plasma.

How safe are large doses of vitamin C? Vitamin C is listed as a GRAS substance, which means it's *generally recognized as safe*. Vitamin C is non-toxic and there are no reported cases of a fatality caused by consumption of any amount of vitamin C. As much as 200,000 milligrams have been taken orally over a period of few hours with no harmful effects. 150,000 milligrams of sodium ascorbate has been given intravenously without problems. A caution with using vitamins is that care must be used taking them when combined with minerals. Do not attempt to increase your vitamin intake by taking vitamin/mineral combinations. Excess ingestion of minerals can be harmful to your health.

The contrast between vitamin C's toxicity and that of a commonly used drug like aspirin could not be clearer. Sixty to 90 tablets of aspirin (20,000 milligrams to 30,000 milligrams) can kill an adult and much less will kill a child. Aspirin is the most common substance used in suicides in the U.S. and 15% of all accidental poisonings of children are caused by aspirin.

Many studies were done in the 1970s allegedly proving that Linus Pauling's advocacy of vitamin C was wrong headed and bad science. Almost all of them used nutritional doses of vitamin C (amounts too low to have significant effects) as opposed to pharmacological doses. The problem with getting good scientific research done on vitamin C is that vitamin C can't be patented so Big Pharma can't make any money from it. If anything, the pharmaceutical industry wishes vitamin C could be regulated or banned outright.

Recently however, a ten year study involving 300,000 men and women, the Finnish-Harvard study, showed that taking 700 milligrams daily cut the risk of death from heart disease by 25%. Yet, the Required Daily Amount is only 60 milligrams. As Linus Pauling once mentioned, it's the first 250 milligrams, not the last 250 milligrams of vitamin C, that are the most important. I find I can easily use 4,000 to 8,000 milligrams for my own personal dose. I also find the *sodium ascorbate* seems to be absorbed easier by my bowels than ascorbic acid. I, like Linus Pauling, think Bronson Pharmaceuticals is a high caliber vitamin company. (My intention in writing this book isn't to sell you vitamins, but to make complex and technical health matters as interesting as I can to reach a wide audience. I have a simple philosophy: The greatest good for the largest number of people, for the least cost.)

What Research Has Shown

Linus Pauling would have loved to see the results of the recent Harvard-Finnish Study, showing the 24% decrease in heart disease mortality due to vitamin C. In 1992, shortly before Pauling passed away, he co-published with Dr. Mathias Rath perhaps the most controversial paper of his long and productive career, titled, "A unified theory of human cardiovascular disease leading to the abolition of this disease as a cause for human mortality." Dr. Mathias Rath also published his book in 1999, *Why Animals Don't Get Heart Disease, But People Do.* Surprisingly, Pauling and Rath weren't the first players in this field.

The first scientist to publish on the subject of vitamin C and heart disease was Canadian biologist J.C. Paterson who published research in 1940 demonstrating that atherosclerosis, heart disease, and damage to artery walls were all caused by a deficiency in vitamin C. He thought from his research that blood clots implicated in strokes were caused by damage to the capillaries in the area of arterial plaques. He measured vitamin C levels in these stroke patients and found them to be very low, stating, "There is sufficient evidence to warrant the recommendation those patients with coronary artery disease be assured an adequate vitamin C intake, either by a proper diet or by the exhibition of ascorbic acid, an innocuous drug."

Another Canadian, Dr. C. G. Willis, followed up Paterson's work and supported his hypothesis that atherosclerosis was caused by deficiencies of vitamin C. He showed that in patients with scurvy, fat was deposited in the artery wall, and he noted that fragile capillaries and lesions would occur at sites where mechanical stress occurred. Their work was confirmed by Dr. Louis J. Ignarro who won a 1998 Nobel Prize in medicine for his studies in nitric oxide signaling in the cardiovascular system. Ignarro found that anti-oxidant vitamins (like vitamin C) and an amino acid, L-arginine, could prevent blood vessel inflammation and subsequent damage to the artery walls in mice.

Despite this research done over 50 years ago suggesting heart disease and atherosclerosis is caused by vitamin deficiencies, the leading textbook for cardiologists, *The Heart—Textbook of Cardiovascular Medicine* by Eugene Braunwald, doesn't mention vitamin C even once in over 2,000 pages!

As I mentioned earlier, heart disease is almost completely unknown in the animal kingdom, primarily because most animals manufacture ample quantities of vitamin C in their liver or kidneys. As long ago as 1958, one of the leading textbooks of veterinary medicine written by T.C. Jones and H. A. Smith stated: "… in none of the domestic species, with the rarest of exceptions, do animals develop atherosclerotic disease of clinical significance. It appears that … atherosclerotic disease in them is not impossible; *it just does not occur.* If the reason for this could be found it might cast some very useful light on the human disease."

Indeed. Here's some "useful light" I'm casting: The largest difference between humans and almost all other species, other than brain capacity, is the tremendous difference in our blood plasma levels of vitamin C. Our levels are between 10 and 100 times lower than most other creatures. Even house flies can manufacture their own vitamin C, but we humans can't make a single molecule. Could high levels of vitamin C in blood plasma in animals explain why they don't develop heart disease?

Taking the vitamin C/heart disease link further, it offers an explanation to the French Paradox, explaining why the French have such lower rates of heart disease than Americans, despite consuming substantially more fat in their rich diet. The reason why is that they have much higher levels of vitamin C due to eating fresh produce, more fruits, organ meats, and fresher foods. It should be noted also the French eat higher quality fats, such as butter instead of margarine, and have more B vitamins in their diet. These are the scientific reasons why French heart disease rates are so low, compared to the popular press notions that consuming wine or olive oil is what makes for healthy French hearts.

It's been well documented that the further north you go in Europe, the higher the rate of heart disease and stroke, and the lower the levels of vitamin C in the blood. The further south you go—despite people eating diets high in saturated fat and being overweight—the lower the levels of heart disease and the higher the levels of vitamin C in the blood.

Forget about the brainwashing you've had all your life about cholesterol or the absurd TV ads stating that cholesterol levels have something to do with your diet or your genetic ancestry. It's perfectly normal for healthy adults to have cholesterol levels of 220 or 240 or even higher. As I mentioned in Chapter Three, a family history of cardiovascular disease is probably due the genetic need (by about 15% of the population) of much higher levels of B vitamins than the average person.

Important Factors Involving Vitamin Needs

The vitamin dose recommendations in the last chapter and in this chapter so far are for prevention and maintenance of good cardiovascular health. A few other factors involving your body's needs for vitamins should be mentioned before we get into dosage amounts and recommendations to reverse existing atherosclerosis and heart disease.

Many diuretic drugs used by millions of people can also greatly increase your risk for cardiovascular disease. Coffee is, of course, a widely used diuretic. Along with the water diuretic drugs flush from your body, essential nutrients and water soluble vitamins are also flushed out. If you're taking diuretic drugs you need to take substantially more vitamins to make up for the loss. Also, all synthetic chemical drugs consumed have to be detoxified by your liver before they can be eliminated from your body. This process uses up vitamin C and many other essential nutrients. Long term use of synthetic chemical drugs leads to chronic vitamin depletion and can cause cardiovascular disease.

It's a good idea to consult a qualified health care practitioner for advice on what levels of vitamins to take. Obviously, you have to ask the right questions to get the right answers. Most medical doctors have little or no education in nutrition or in prescribing vitamins and minerals. Also, if you're currently under treatment for cardiovascular disease you need to tell your doctor what vitamins and minerals or anti-oxidants you're taking as they may have inter-actions with chemical drugs.

Remember: vitamins are safe—drugs are not.

Reversing Heart Disease with Vitamins and Minerals

Here's the vitamin therapy recommended by Linus Pauling and Mathias Rath, from *Ascorbate, The Science of Vitamin C* by Steve Hickey PhD and Hillary Roberts, for curing atherosclerosis and coronary heart disease:

NUTRITIONAL SUPPLEMENTS	DAILY AMOUNT IN GRAMS (Split into 3 doses)
Vitamin C	3-6 (3,000 to 6,000 mg)
Lysine	3-6 (3,000 to 6,000 mg)
Proline	0.5-2 (500 to 2,000 mg)

The rationale behind the use of lysine and proline, two amino acids which are found in large quantities in meat, is they have synergistic effects with vitamin C to reverse hardening of the arteries. The amino acid proline acts like Teflon, helping to neutralize the stickiness of fat globules (lipoproteins) in your arteries. Proline helps to prevent more atherosclerotic deposits from occurring and to release already deposited lipoproteins. Proline is a major building block of the proteins collagen and elastin that are needed in quantity to build strong artery walls. Your body can manufacture proline, but not in the quantities needed to help repair damaged arteries.

Lysine is an essential amino acid and your body cannot synthesize it. It also is a building block for collagen and also has Teflon-like qualities for removing atherosclerotic deposits. Both of these substances are natural, and unlike chemical drugs, are of very low toxicity.

If you have heart disease and want to take a powerful full spectrum vitamin and Mineral formula to reverse your cardiovascular disease, I recommend you take Dr. Mathias Rath's patented formulas. You can research them on the Internet (www.drrathvitamins.com), or buy them through your local heath food store. His formula is probably the best you can buy.

I have included the basic formula recommended by Linus Pauling and reported in *Ascorbate, The Science of Vitamin C*, because it's cheap, harmless, and can be done by those who can't afford medical treatment (or even expensive vitamin formulas) for their existing heart disease. *The Santa Barbara Diet* is a book written with a global audience in mind. Not everyone can afford the high tech schemes and "solutions" for heart disease offered by modern medicine. As always, an ounce of prevention is better than a pound of cure.

Another formula mentioned in *Ascorbate, The Science of Vitamin C* is the Anti-Oxidant Network Therapy Formula, as shown below:

ANTI-OXIDANT NETWORK THERAPY FORMULA	
Vitamin C	At or Near Bowel Tolerance, 6 + grams
Lysine	3-6 grams.
Proline	5-2 grams
Natural vitamin E	800 I.U. units (Only use d-alpha tocopherol)
R-Lipoic Acid	300 to 600 milligrams

These supplements should be split into three doses and the vitamin regimen should be taken between two months to as long as two years, to achieve desired results.

Because of the rigors of the scientific method, I won't tell you this vitamin regimen is curative. It's the sort of harmless vitamin program that needs good studies to be done, to prove or disprove its efficacy. Of course, along with this program you need to make sure you are taking adequate amounts of magnesium, as it is the most important mineral for your heart. As mentioned earlier in the book, one must be careful taking magnesium if you have kidney disease. Check with your physician to make sure you don't have kidney problems that could interact with increased magnesium intake.

If you are at risk for heart disease and choose to use the Pauling/Rath vitamin formula to reverse heart disease or the Anti-Oxidant Network formula, keep in mind that when you first start upon a vitamin program to reverse the hardening of your arteries and to remove arterial plaque, you might see a rise in your cholesterol levels. This temporary rise is a sign of the healing process of your artery walls and of the decrease in fatty deposits. You should continue your vitamin treatments a few months past when your cholesterol levels decline lower than they were when you started.

Here's some dietary tips: Adding barley, oat bran, oatmeal and increased fiber to your diet will greatly aid the process. Eating an apple daily is also an excellent boost to your dietary fiber. A little known fact is that barley is more effective than oatmeal for helping lower cholesterol levels. A good way to eat barley is to buy pressed barley ("oshi mugi") at your local Japanese or Asian Market and cook it the same way you'd cook oatmeal. Soak it overnight with an equal amount of water, before cooking it, the same way you should cook oatmeal. Adding up to a tablespoon of lemon or lime juice or whey when soaking, will add to the nutritional value of the barley.

Ending Note

Linus Pauling suggested his vitamin therapy would *cure* heart disease and hardening of the arteries. However, the medical establishment doesn't like to use the word *cure*. Obviously, curing a chronic condition with low cost, safe vitamin supplements is not in the best interests of the global pharmaceutical and medical industries.

Probably, the best thing I could say to you in closing this chapter about vitamin C, are the words with which Linus Pauling ended his book, *How to Live Longer and Feel Better*, written in 1986: "Do not let the medical authorities or the politicians mislead you. Find out what the facts are, and make your own decisions about how to live a happy life and how to work for a better world."

CHAPTER FIVE

Sugar —
Public Enemy Number One

In the summer of 2006, I attended the 4th of July parade in Lander, Wyoming and watched the float of the Eastern Shoshone Tribal Diabetes Clinic roll down Main Street. I couldn't help but notice that, like many of the spectators, the Native Americans on the floats were big people. As their colorful float passed by, and the Shoshones on board were busily throwing candy to the crowd, a loud announcement came from the bandstand telling us all that federal funding for the new Dialysis Center had just been approved. Watching the kids running to snatch up the candy, I wondered if anyone besides me made the connection between those sugar candies bouncing on the pavement and the very avoidable disease of diabetes.

The Sugar Disease

For the people who have diabetes or will get diabetes, you need to know the most common form, *type 2 diabetes*, happens because of the choices you make. Type 2 diabetes is a life style disease—you choose it or you avoid it—it's entirely up to you. If you allow yourself to become addicted to sugar, you'll walk the diabetes path until your limbs are amputated, you go blind, or your heart fails. First the crutch, then the wheelchair, then you go blind—then your heart fails. Those are the steps along the path of getting diabetes, the Sugar Disease. Not a pretty picture, is it?

Hopefully, this chapter will change the way you think about sugar for the rest of your life. When it comes to sugar, ignorance is not bliss. Trust me—it would not be fun rolling around in a wheelchair after your legs have been amputated. Diabetes also makes you go blind or causes your vision to fail. You might even need to have your wheelchair pushed up close to the TV, so you can keep watching your favorite shows. Not to mention, it might be hard to support yourself when you're dealing with massive medical bills or dialysis treatments. If you're lucky, Uncle Sugar—I mean Uncle Sam—might still be there to pick up the tab. But, I wouldn't count on it; relying on the benevolence of strangers, especially tall skinny guys from Washington, D.C., isn't usually the best strategy in life.

In talking about sugar and diabetes, we want to distinguish between the two different types of diabetes. A very small number of both children and adults have type 1 diabetes, which used to be called *juvenile-onset diabetes,* because it usually develops in childhood. Type 1 diabetes is less than 5 to 10% of all cases and occurs because the immune system (for unknown reasons) kills off cells in your pancreas needed to make *insulin,* an important hormone that metabolizes *glucose,* your body's primary fuel. Type 2 diabetes, which I'm calling the Sugar Disease, is different. Type 2 is the kind of diabetes that's causing the epidemic of the century, turning millions of people in affluent countries all over the world into helpless cripples.

Type 2 diabetes occurs because of the consumption of excess amounts of dietary sugar, which is really an unnatural chemical product called *sucrose.* Excessive amounts of sucrose interacts with hydrogenated oils and trans-fats in our modern diet, causing the body's muscle and liver tissues to lose their ability to metabolize that important hormone *insulin.* To compensate, the cells in your pancreas crank out higher and higher levels of insulin, until eventually they die of exhaustion. The end result is similar to what happens in type 1 diabetes: your body can no longer metabolize glucose, its most important primary fuel. And that's when things start falling apart.

Because of the massive increase in the amount of sugar as sucrose and corn syrup being consumed by Americans, type 2 diabetes, which used to only occur in people older than 40, is now occurring at a much younger age. Between 1990 and 2001, diabetes type 2 cases have almost doubled among people between people 30 to 50 years old. Cases have also increased by 50% among people between age 18 and 29. This is an alarming trend.

The connection between commercial sugar and obesity in the diabetes epidemic is as solid as the links in a steel chain. A 25 year long study of nurses showed that obese people were 40 times (!) more likely to develop diabetes than those of normal weight. Some researchers believe that people with big bellies are more likely to develop diabetes because of biochemicals spewed out by large fat deposits in the liver and the abdomen. The exact mechanism isn't completely understood.

Currently, 18 million Americans have been diagnosed with type 2 diabetes. The latest estimates are that over 40 million Americans have pre-diabetes, which means their blood sugar levels are high enough to indicate they will probably get diabetes unless they choose to change their ways. If you don't already have diabetes, it can be easily avoided by making a few simple changes in your life. There is a simple, inexpensive remedy, and it's actually fun. You only have to eliminate excessive sugar from your diet and do the simple exercise routine mentioned at the end of this chapter.

Sugar, Obesity, and other Defective Foods

I would be seriously remiss in not mentioning the connection between obesity and a particularly dangerous and defective form of dietary sugar, *high fructose corn syrup*. Between 1985 and 1995, the total amount of sucrose (chemical, commercial sugar) consumed increased every year, but the lion's share of the increase was high fructose corn syrup and dextrose (corn sugar).

After 1995, sugar consumption flattened out because of the large increase in non-caloric chemicals, such as *aspartame,* marketed as NutraSweet and used to replace sugar. Chemical sweeteners have their own set of problems that I'll go over later in this chapter. There's only one magic bullet in the world of sugar substitutes—it's called *stevia*. It's safe to use and has almost no calories. More about stevia later...

The huge rise in consumption of high fructose corn syrup, as it steadily replaced sugar (sucrose) in many soft drinks, can only exacerbate America's diabetes problem. About 800 million bushels of corn are now grown in America each year to produce high fructose corn syrup for American's food industry. Leave it to America's junk food manufacturers to come up with a new menace to your health that's probably worse for you than sugar.

Recent experiments at the University of Cincinnati showed mice that drank high fructose corn syrup instead of water appeared to have their metabolism altered in a way that favored fat storage. They ate less food, gained more weight, and put on 90% more body fat than mice that drank only water. Conclusion: The high fructose corn syrup that makes you fat, also makes you vulnerable to type 2 diabetes.

I hope that what I'm writing isn't too disturbing and controversial to those of you who've been lifelong consumers of the many defective foods manufactured by America's agri-business and junk food industries. After all, manufacturing them is the largest business in America. These businesses sell over $1 trillion of product each year.

Before these food industries gained such control of the food supply, diseases such as diabetes and heart disease were almost unknown. Their increase parallels the rise in the use of sugar, processed foods, canned foods, white flour, hydrogenated oils, oxidized cholesterols, margarine and other faux foods. The average per capita consumption of sugar in 1821 was only ten pounds. Consequently, in the 19th century diabetes was extremely rare, as was cancer and heart disease. In 1900, the Metropolitan Life Insurance Company compiled a list of the causes of death, and diabetes was 27th on the list. By 1950, it had climbed up the charts to be the 3rd leading cause of death.

Currently in America, the average annual consumption of sugar is between 160 and 180 pounds per person. This amount is about 45% sucrose and 55% high fructose corn syrup and dextrose (corn sugar). In 1986, Linus Pauling wrote in his book, *How to Live Longer and Feel Better*, that in order to be healthy, one should consume less than 50 pounds of sugar annually.

At the time Pauling wrote, the average annual consumption was only 100 lbs. Hmmmm; do you think there might be a correlation between this rise in sugar consumption and the rise in diabetes? Since sugar, sold commercially as sucrose, isn't found anywhere in nature, your might want to pay close attention to the words of a two time Nobel Prize winner, and the most important chemist of the last 100 years, when he cautions you to eat less than 50 lbs annually of sugar.

Rene Dubos, famed French micro-biologist and humanist, once said about Linus Pauling: "The future catches up with Pauling 20 years later...." For those of you who didn't grow up in the Roaring Sixties, Rene Dubos is mostly remembered now for coining the phrase, *Think globally and act locally.*

military industrial complex, and doing early research on using electric cars, for stating the benefits of vitamin C and exposing the dangers of tobacco—and sugar. Last but not least—*Sugar*!

Some Facts and Lies About Sugar

I realize in writing this story that many people are confused by the different types of sugars and how your body reacts to them. This is what you need to know: *Fructose* is fruit sugar, *maltose* is malt sugar, *lactose* is milk sugar, *dextrose* is corn sugar, and *sucrose* (commonly called sugar) is a highly refined sugar made from sugar cane and sugar beets. I'll give you information on the chemical sugar substitute Splenda and the deadly neuro-toxin *aspartame* further on down the slippery, sweet path.

Many food manufacturers and producers label sugar as a carbohydrate, a practice that is deliberately misleading. Since the labeling requirements came out on foods, refined carbohydrates such as sugar are lumped together with other carbohydrates that may or may not have been refined. Refined and unrefined, all are added together for a carbohydrate total. The effect of this process is to hide the sugar content from you, the food purchaser.

Another trick is to break down the sugar content on the label into high fructose corn syrup, dextrose, maltose, etc. to keep from having to list "sugar" as the primary ingredient in a food. Many of the processed foods sold in America have three primary ingredients: sugar, white flour and hydrogenated oil. Look closely at labels and you'll see food manufacturers can make almost anything from combinations of these Big Three ingredients. Sugar is often the primary ingredient in hundreds of food products sold in American grocery stores.

Another common trick is to use the words *glucose* or *sucrose* interchangeably. Glucose is a natural sugar found with other sugars in fruits and vegetables. Many of the foods you eat are converted into glucose in your body. In fact, the term glucose is used is to refer to sugar that is carried by your blood, more commonly, blood sugar.

Be careful not to confuse *glucose* with *sucrose*, a man-made chemical. Glucose is a key component in the metabolism of all animals and plants. It has always been an essential element in the human bloodstream. On the other hand, sucrose (sugar) and our 20th century addiction to it is something quite new to the human animal. Our ancient genes have evolved over millions of years, and they've only been exposed to sugar on a large scale for less than 200 years.

Over the last 200 years, most of the natural sugars in our diet have been replaced by sucrose or high fructose corn syrup. This is done by the process of taking a natural food containing high percentages of fruit or vegetable sugar and removing all other elements until only the sugar remains. Sucrose, or white sugar, is made by taking sugar cane or sugar beets and pressing them until all the juice is removed. This juice is then heated and lime is added. Moisture is removed through a vacuum process, and then the crystals are run through a centrifuge. The solution is then boiled and passed through a series of charcoal filters. Then the sugar is bleached snow white with extracts from cattle bones. As many as 64 different food elements are destroyed in the refining process, including potassium, magnesium, calcium, iron, sulfate and sodium, along with vital enzymes, amino acids and all of the vitamins.

While "white" refined sugar is not natural to your body, your body has no problem using natural sugars such as those found in honey, maple syrup, brown rice syrup, agave syrup, birch syrup, or fructose, the natural sugar found in fruit. Of these natural sugars, fructose is probably the finest, healthiest, and most beneficial sugar you can consume. Natural fruit sugars like fructose are processed so easily by your body, they don't even require digestion. In your liver, they're converted into glucose to be available for your body's energy needs, or they are stored in your liver as glycogen for later use.

Sugar: A Deadly Habit

High sugar consumption robs your body of what it needs for health and eventually kills you. When you eat a highly refined carbohydrate like sugar, your body must take nutrients from healthy cells to metabolize the sugar. Sugar as we buy it commercially is a toxic chemical substance that depletes your supplies of potassium, magnesium, sodium, and calcium as sugar is excreted from your body.

the sugar habit is a process not unlike what drug addicts go through. Millions have chosen to kick the habit and you too, can succeed if you chose to do so.

Sugar is probably the deadliest substance ever ingested by humans in large quantities. It's been linked by good research over the last 70 years to heart disease, kidney failure, liver disease, diabetes, hyperactivity, and atherosclerosis. Sugar is also strongly associated with cancer in test animals and humans. Cancerous tumors are also known to be large absorbers of sugar. A good reason to cut back on your sugar consumption is that cancer cells consume more than 18 times as much as sugar as normal cells. Everyone has some cancer cells in their body at all times (see Chapter 8) and eating sugar is a good way to encourage their growth.

One of the early sugar researchers, whose work was noted by Linus Pauling, was pioneer researcher, John Yudkin, a professor of physiology, nutrition, and dietetics. His best known book, *Sweet and Dangerous*, was published in 1972. In 1957, he published studies of death rates from 15 countries correlating coronary heart disease and sugar consumption. The annual rate per 100,000 people goes like this:

- ✓ 60 will die each year from consuming 20 pounds of sugar.
- ✓ 300 will die each year from consuming 120 pounds of sugar.
- ✓ 750 will die each year consuming 150 pounds of sugar.

We've now reached the point where close to 24% of the calories consumed in America are from sugar. Alcohol is, of course, another beverage with high sugar content. Alcohol consumption accounts for as much of 10% of total calories consumed in America.

Marketing Sugar and Sugar Substitutes: Big Business

Sugar is big business, both in its unnatural forms as sucrose and high fructose corn syrup and in chemical sugar substitutes that are usually worse for you than what they are replacing.

The food processing industry loves sucrose/sugar because it has a long shelf life, adds taste and sweetness to junk foods, and also prevents foods from spoiling. Additionally, America's sugar growers received 465 million dollars in the year 2000 *not* to grow sugar. In turn, these producers spend large amounts of money on political payola to keep import quotas on foreign produced sugar to prevent it from entering the U.S. market. It's estimated those quotas cost American consumers more than $2 billion annually in higher prices. As if the health consequences of sugar production wasn't enough, the sugar industry collects subsidies, uses the political process to ban cheaper foreign production, and continually attempts to outlaw or ban natural, healthy sugar substitutes, such as the herb stevia.

The most profitable drug delivery vehicle for sugar has always been soda pop. Until the recent marketing of synthetic chemical drugs, such as the cholesterol lowering statins, Coca-Cola and Pepsi have been among the most profitable products in the history of the U.S. They contribute nothing to your diet except a momentary sugar buzz, and they can leave you with life long health problems. Not to worry—*It's the Real Thing*—and *Things Go Better with Pepsi!*

Among the other problems (besides sugar) with Pepsi and Coke is they're extremely high in phosphoric acid. The use of Coke and Pepsi are well documented contributors to our nation's osteoporosis epidemic, also. The pH of Coke is 2.8, and it will dissolve a nail in about four days. Hmmmm, what does that stuff do to your bones? I think both Coke and Pepsi should have a skull and crossbones symbol on their labels as a consumer warning. In a different way, they're as deleterious to your health as tobacco or hard liquor.

QUICK TIPS FOR USING THE COKE/PEPSI YOU'RE NO LONGER DRINKING

To clean the toilet: Pour a can of Coke into the toilet bowl and let "The Real Thing" sit for one hour, then flush clean. The citric acid in Coke removes stains from vitreous china.

To clean battery terminals: Pour Coke or Pepsi over the crusty terminals to bubble away corrosion.

To remove rust from auto bumpers: Rub the bumper with a crumpled piece of Reynolds aluminum foil dipped in Coca-Cola.

stains from asphalt after an accident.

Millions of Americans have cut down on the sugar consumed in sugary beverages like soda pop by drinking Diet-Coke and other products that are designed to be low in calories. Unfortunately, these low calorie sweeteners have their own set of problems. Linus Pauling stated flatly in 1986, "I do not recommend the diet sodas, in which the sucrose is replaced by artificial sweeteners, because I am worried about the possible toxicity of these non orthomolecular substances." At the time he was referring to Saccharine which has been used for a long time as a chemical sweetener despite its link to cancer in test animals and humans

Currently, the largest source of health complaints to the FDA come from the use of a product first developed by the G. D. Searle Company called *aspartame.* You probably know it by its product names of NutraSweet or Equal. Selling you NutraSweet is very big business indeed, and it has helped keep the great bandwagon rolling for defective, dangerous products like Coca-Cola and Pepsi. They've been able to avoid their link to sugar and give you a "healthy" option of still using their products but not getting any calories or sugar. The rather obvious problem is that one can of Coke or Pepsi has about 10 teaspoons of sugar and 140 to 150 nutritionally empty calories

The story of how aspartame/NutraSweet was approved for mass consumption is a Washington-style version of the movie *Chinatown.* Donald Rumsfield, the recently retired head of the U.S. Department of Defense and one of the chief planners of the failed occupation of Iraq, was the much feared CEO of G. D. Searle in the late 1970s and the prime mover in getting aspartame approved.

Aspartame was first discovered in 1966 by a research scientist at G. D. Searle who was trying to develop an ulcer drug. It was developed as a sugar substitute after the scientist accidentally licked his fingers and discovered they tasted sweet. Aspartame is an rDNA derivative that's made of amino acids. At one time, it was listed as a prospective chemical warfare weapon on a list submitted to Congress by the Pentagon.

Aspartame is made of three components: aspartic acid, phenylalanine, and methanol amino acids saturated in petrochemicals. When it's ingested, it breaks down into its amino acids and methanol, which then biodegrades into *formaldehyde*, the chemical used to embalm corpses. Monsanto, one of the leading manufacturers of aspartame, says: "Formaldehyde has been implicated as a possible carcinogen when inhaled, but this hasn't been shown to be the case when taken by mouth." I guess it doesn't matter to the pickled corpses!

What's wrong with aspartame? Besides breaking down into formaldehyde in your body, aspartame also breaks down into *aspartate*, which is an excitatory amino acid (EAA). Ingesting too many EAAs will kill neurons in your brain. Children's brain cells are more susceptible than adults to die from an overload of EAAs. Published studies done with laboratory animals have clearly shown consuming aspartame can cause the death of brain cells in the hypothalamus. Why should you care about your hypothalamus? Among other reasons, you should care, is because it controls your appetite and sensations involving eating. In a recent issue of *Neurotoxicology*, Dr. John Olney stated animals don't show the effects of hypothalamic damage immediately. The problems surface later on and they include obesity, alterations in the onset of puberty, and infertility. Does this sound like a movie coming to a town near where you live?

Sugar is bad for you, but at least it's not a toxic neuro-chemical like aspartame. Aspartame alters the serotonin balance in your brain, decreases the hypothalamus neuropeptide NPY, and changes norepinephrine concentrations. There are over 90 reported dangerous side effects of aspartame in scientific literature. It can produce brain tumors, lead to blindness, cause memory loss, and chronic fatigue. Aspartame is a neuro-toxin that's been linked to grand mal seizures, brain cancer and central nervous system disorders.

Industry-sponsored research that tested aspartate on monkeys showed there were no ill effects from excitatory amino acids (EAAs). There was one minor detail left out of this research in the summary and conclusions. They didn't mention that the monkeys used in these experiments were kept anesthetized during these aspartate experiments. *And that the type of anesthesia used—phencyclidine—blocks the pathway the chemicals take in order to kill hypothalamus cells.* It's not avoided by the research parameters

Judging from these experiments, are soft drinks with aspartame safe for you and your children to drink? Absolutely! As long as you're anesthetized at all times like the test monkeys, with phencyclidine anesthesia! Otherwise, you should play it safe and drink 100% fruit juices or water.

Sweet Politics: Rumsfield's Coup

How did such a seriously defective product like aspartame ever get approved by the FDA? The answer, of course, lies in the enormous amounts of money to be made by getting a non-caloric sweetener approved by the FDA.

G. D. Searle Company, owner of the manufacturing rights to aspartame, first tried to get aspartame approved in 1973, and an independent scientific board reviewed the evidence and turned it down as being unsafe. G. D. Searle did, however manage to get it approved in 1974 for restricted use in a dry form. Some independent scientists raised questions (do we have any of those independent scientists left?), and an FDA investigation was launched to scrutinize Searle's data. What they found was a real eye-opener. Searle's own data showed that of seven infant monkeys that had received aspartame in their milk, one had died and five others had grand mal seizures. Somehow (oops!), this data had been left out of Searle's first application.

In 1977, the U.S. Attorney General's office received a request from the FDA to investigate Searle for making false claims and for concealing data in their tests of aspartame. The U.S. Attorney General's office didn't follow through on this complaint and when the statute of limitations ran out, the matter was dropped. Lots of other things weren't going too well for Searle & Company in 1977. Their stock had dropped from $110 per share to $12 and earnings had dropped by 23%.

The Searle Company was based in the Chicago area and despite their troubles, was still one of the country's most prominent pharmaceutical manufacturers with patents on Dramamine, the motion sickness drug, and Enovid, an early birth control pill. Searle was also located in the district of former Illinois congressman, Donald Rumsfield, who had recently retired as Secretary of Defense in the Ford administration. The G. D. Searle Company knew Rumsfield well, as they had contributed money to Rumsfield's first campaign, when he ran for Congress. In 1977, they hired Donald Rumsfield to take over as Chief Executive Officer.

Rumsfield quickly showed he could translate the "take no prisoners" management style he'd used in the federal government into the world of business. Within nine months, he had divested 20 unprofitable businesses and cut Searle's corporate staff from 800 employees down to 350. Stories were circulated of employees paged at airports, asked to come home, and fired on the spot. Within a few years, Rumsfield had been included in a list by *Fortune Magazine* of the "10 toughest bosses" in American business.

In 1979, the FDA certified a Board of Public Enquiry to investigate the safety issues surrounding aspartame. The determination of the board was there is no "proof of reasonable certainty that aspartame is safe as a food additive."

Being a lifelong Republican, Rumsfield was overjoyed when Ronald Reagan came to power in 1980, and he was on the transition team helping the Reaganites take office. According to a former G. D. Searle salesperson quoted from the Internet, "Rumsfield said in a sales meeting that he would call in all his markers, and no matter what, he would see to it that aspartame would be approved that year."

One day after Ronald Reagan was inaugurated in 1981, Searle reapplied (without any new data or tests) for approval of aspartame. The new head of the FDA, Arthur Hayes, was involved in empanelling another advisory board to determine the safety of aspartame, and as a result, an in-house panel once again recommended against approving aspartame.

Around that time, the National Soft Drink Association even lobbied the FDA not to approve NutraSweet. Their opposition was primarily based upon the fact that when aspartame is heated above 86 degrees, it breaks down into a poison called free methanol (wood alcohol). This is a problem, because when heated to 98.6 degrees (what temperature is your body?), it breaks down further into formic acid (used to strip epoxy) and formaldehyde (embalming fluid.)

However, despite all this commotion, in 1981 the new head of the FDA, Arthur Hayes, overruled the Public Board of Enquiry, ignored the recommendations of his own FDA staff, and approved NutraSweet for dry products. In 1983, Hayes granted FDA approval for use of aspartame in carbonated beverages. Within four months, Hayes left the FDA and took a lucrative job in G. D. Searle's public relations firm as a senior medical consultant.

Currently, aspartame (the largest sales come under the trademarked names of Equal and NutraSweet) is the basis of over 75% of all consumer complaints to the Food and Drug Administration. There are at least five reported deaths attributed to aspartame. In the first Gulf War, some of the troops of Desert Storm were exposed to aspartame sweetened sodas which had been left out in the Saudi Arabian heat and sunlight on pallet loads. Many of the troops who drank these beverages returned home with disorders similar to those of people poisoned by formaldehyde. The free methanol in the beverages may have been a factor in these illnesses.

But where there's money to be made, the food industry in America always keeps moving on. As legendary sandlot baseball pitcher Satchel Paige once observed—"Don't look back—something might be gaining on you!"

Splenda vs. Stevia

The newest kid strutting his stuff down Sugar Street is Splenda, the commercial name for yet another artificial sugar substitute. At the present time, the market for Splenda, the newest non-caloric sweetener, is booming. It's taken over 50% of the market share of the over $500 million annual business of low calorie sweeteners. Like its predecessors made from aspartame, Splenda is causing a large number of complaints with the FDA regarding its safety.

The marketing spin on this new product is that it's safer than the other products of the past, such as Sweet and Low, Equal and NutraSweet. It's made from sugar—so it's safe (or so they say)—yet it has no calories. The Sugar Association is currently suing manufacturer McNeil Nutritionals over their claim that Splenda is made from sugar.

Made from sugar, so it tastes like sugar is the central campaign of the marketing program.

Monica Neufang, a spokesperson for McNeil Nutritionals, said the false advertising claims filed by the Sugar Association are without merit. She refused to disclose how much McNeil spends annually on advertising and said the company has never represented the product as being natural. She was quoted in the *Wall Street Journal* as saying "We start the process of making Splenda with sugar. There are trucks full of sugar that pull up outside of our plant."

If you've followed my train of thought in this chapter, you realize the complete absurdity of anyone calling, or implying sugar is a natural product. Sugar starts out as a natural product until it's refined into a chemically pure substance which has less than zero nutritional value. That's natural? The implication that sugar is natural or good for you is a brazen lie.

The FDA has no definition for "natural" anyway, so whether it's "natural or "made from sugar" is irrelevant. Splenda is the trade name for *sucralose*, a synthetic chemical compound discovered in 1976 in England by scientists seeking new pesticide formulas. It's true that the Splenda molecule is made up of sugar, except that three of the hydroxyl groups in the molecule have been replaced by chlorine atoms. Industry experts claim the resulting molecule is similar to table salt or sugar, but other independent researchers say it has more in common with the molecular structure of many pesticides. This is because the bonds holding the carbon and chlorine atoms are more characteristic of a chlorocarbon than a salt, and most pesticides are chlorocarbons. Technically speaking, sucralose (Splenda) is a chlorinated sucrose derivative that is also combined with dextrose (corn sugar) and maltodextrin (a drying agent).

I can't guarantee that something containing chlorine atoms or that might be similar in structure to pesticides is safe or isn't. But why would you want your family to be human guinea pigs or test monkeys for this new experiment? Of course, because of the money to be made, Splenda was rushed through the FDA approval processes without any thorough, long-term, independent investigation.

Splenda is designed like the synthetic faux fat Olestra, manufactured by Proctor and Gamble and approved by the FDA in 1998, to be a substance that your body doesn't recognize as food. That's why it has no calories. In theory, when it gets into your stomach and your intestines, your body excretes it. However, some recent FDA tests show that as much as 11 to 27% of Splenda is absorbed by your body. The Japanese Sanitation Council did tests showing as much as 40% was absorbed. Does the idea of ingesting chlorinated molecules of a new chemical substance similar in structure to pesticides into all of your tissues sound like a good idea to you?

On Splenda's official website, the news is being proclaimed that Splenda is safe and has no side effects. It's always Good News Week on Splenda's website! Thank you McNeil Nutritionals for sponsoring the bake sales at our schools and giving away all those tasty Splenda recipes! Also, special thanks to Tate and Lyle, PLC, the London based company that supplies the wonderful sugar that Splenda is made from.

I don't need to go over the many side effects and allergic reactions that thousands of people are having from ingesting chlorinated Splenda molecules into their systems. If you've ever used this product, you should Google it on the Internet and look over the many sites where unhappy consumers are commiserating about their symptoms from using Splenda. Given the sordid story of NutraSweet/aspartame, I'm not holding my breath for the FDA to do anything in the interest of the public health. Nor should you. Just stop eating it!

Consider instead using natural sweets such as honey, maple syrup, brown rice syrup, agave syrup, and many other natural sugars. If you desire to use a low calorie sweetener, you should use *stevia*.

For those of you who haven't heard of stevia, it's a plant native to Paraguay in South America and has been used by the Guárani Indians for centuries. It's a natural herb that has zero calories, is 250 to 300 times sweeter than sugar, and is safe for diabetics. It has a long history of use by humans with no documented problems. You can currently buy stevia as a white powder extracted from the leaves of the plant at your local health food store.

It's worth noting that only because of the legislation enacted in 1994 during the Clinton administration protecting your right to buy vitamins and dietary supplements, can you purchase Stevia at your local health food store or over the Internet. Even though you can purchase it as a dietary supplement, any mention of using it as a sweetener or as an herbal tea is strictly prohibited by the FDA. The Food and Drug Administration has labeled stevia an "unsafe food additive" and has gone to extensive lengths such as a "search and seizure" program and an "import alert" to keep stevia from the U.S. market. Rob McCaleb, the president and founder of the Herb Research Foundation as quoted in *New Age Journal*, summed the situation up, "Sweetness is big money. Nobody wants to see something cheap and easy grow on the market, competing with the things they worked so hard to get approved."

In Japan, stevia has captured over 40% of the market share of the natural sweetener market and has been used extensively in food products since 1970. The Japanese banned dangerous artificial food additives and artificial sweeteners during the 1960s as part of a strong trend not to allow chemical products in their food supply, so their market was ripe for the introduction of stevia. It is currently grown and used widely in Germany, China, Israel, South Korea, and Malaysia.

I started out in this chapter mentioning the hazards of soft drinks to your health, and now I want to link the Sugar Disease, type 2 diabetes, and the profits made by food processing companies as well as pharmaceutical companies. Just think of the money being made as the average American now drinks 52.3 gallons of soda each year. This is in contrast to the average consumption of 20.3 gallons of milk and 16.6 gallons of bottled water for the same time period.

It shouldn't be too surprising to most of us that new research from the Harvard School of Health and a study of 52,000 nurses concluded that the greater amounts of sugar sweetened colas and other sugared drinks consumed were strongly linked to diabetes. Interestingly enough, in an eight year long study, no link was found to diabetes among those who drank 100% fruit juice. But those who drank fruit punches (some fruit juice and a lot of sugar) had double the risk of developing diabetes than a control group. In the study published in the *Journal of the American Medical Association*, the researchers concluded, "We found positive associations between sugar sweetened beverage consumption and both greater weight gain and risk of type 2 diabetes, independent of known risk factors."

Richard Adamson, the American Beverage Society's vice president for scientific and technical affairs, in a follow-up story in the *Wall Street Journal*: "It is inexplicable that the authors have chosen to focus solely on sugar sweetened beverages in this way. Neither soft drinks nor fruit juice consumption nor sugar intake are listed by the National Institutes of Health, the American Diabetic Association or the majority of published literature as risk factors for type 2 diabetes. *This study provides no evidence to support the inflammatory allegation that sugar sweetened beverages are a cause of type 2 diabetes.*"

I should mention that in writing this book, I spent almost three years clipping news stories from the *Wall Street Journal, Fortune, Forbes* and *Barron's.* I quickly realized that in the modern business world, your good health is on the chopping block every day. It's a big mistake thinking the government is doing much of anything to regulate the egregious excesses of Corporate America. Unfortunately, your government has pushed you off the mountain and sold you down the river.....

I'd be remiss in this chapter on sugar and diabetes in not mentioning the second most favored sugar delivery vehicle after soda pop, and that is, of course, breakfast cereals. In 2005, General Mills had the chutzpah to launch a major ad campaign targeted at children, touting the health benefits of breakfast cereal. Some of those "healthy" breakfast cereals were the types they refer to as pre-sweetened, such as Kix, Cocoa Puffs, Cinnamon Toast Crunch, and Count Chocula. General Mills declined to say how much it would spend on its latest ad campaign for pre-sweetened cereals to air on Nickelodeon and the Cartoon Network.

As the diabetes epidemic gathers speed, its estimated over 40 million people in America will be diabetics in the near future and the annual cost for medical bills alone will be over 200 billion dollars. Not to worry—America's biggest drug companies are busy making 'cures' for you. Amylin and its partner Lilly recently won FDA approval for their new drug, Byetta, which mimics a naturally produced hormone that helps regulate glucose. Initially, the twice daily injections might limit sales, but they hope to get a once a week version approved before long.

A recent article on diabetes in *Barron's* had some interesting information on the business of making money from your Sugar Sickness. I quote from the August 15, 2005 issue: "One other experimental drug has wildly excited investors and diabetes doctors. ... Acomplia is a drug that Sanofi-Aventis recently submitted for FDA approval (that) dulls food cravings. Test patients lost nearly 20 pounds over the course of a year. .... If Acomplia is approved ... it will be snapped up by diabetes docs. ... Annual sales of Acomplia could top $5 billion and help Sanofi shares rise from a recent 44 to 51." This article quotes one researcher as saying: "What an opportunity for drug companies! It's a great time to be doing new discovery and diabetes!"

As *The Santa Barbara Diet* was going to press, the process of getting the diet drug Acomplia approved took another surprising turn. An FDA panel unanimously rejected Acomplia because recent drug trials showed it caused depression and "suicidal thinking" in users. It also rejected the drug's name, and if it does get approval, will probably be named Zimulti. This rejection by the panel doesn't mean Acomplia-Zimulti, also known generically as Rimonabant, will be rejected. That final decision will be made by the end of July by the FDA. Recently, the FDA has had more pressure from members of Congress for its lax handling of drug safety issues. The recent findings of the sharply increased risk of heart attacks caused by GlaxoSmithKline diabetes drug Avandia, has caused increased scrutiny of the many dangerous side effects of prescription drugs.

The many problems created by the new non-prescription drug for weight loss, Alli (a non-prescription form of Orlistat/Xenical), that has been flying off the shelves and creating huge profits for GlaxoSmithKline, is yet another all-American, anything-for-a-buck story. One of the side effects of this "fat-blocking" drug is that it can cause the fat to come out of your body in embarrassing ways.

Glaxo's website, myalli.com (isn't that cute and friendly?) warns that Alli can cause you to have gas with oily "discharges" and loose or frequent stools. This site (!) says it's probably a "smart idea" to wear dark clothes and bring a change of clothes to work with you, if you're an Alli user.

I'm mentioning Acomplia and Alli because, if you're a sugar addict and have diabetes, your doctor might prescribe Acomplia, Alli, Orlistat, or Xenical to help you lose weight. Pay close attention to the many side effects of these bizarre chemical concoctions that Big Pharma has cooked up to make a buck from your ignorance and lack of self control. Why not go natural and use my recommendations for fasting to lose weight—see Chapter 9—and gain control of your addictions to fatty foods and sugar!

The Simple Solution

Surprisingly enough, a small amount of diet and exercise can do more to prevent diabetes than anything else you could do. Those who walk half an hour five times each week and lose 7% of their body weight (typically about 15 lbs) can reduce their chance of getting diabetes by 58%—a much better showing than any drug could do for you!

A few final questions: Would you rather eliminate sugar from your diet and take a walk every day? Or would you rather drink soda pop, eat sugary foods, take drugs for the rest of your life, and roll around in a wheelchair after your legs have been amputated? The choice, I hope you now realize, is up to you.

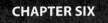
Milk In America: Green Pastures Or Factory Farms?

I grew up in the heart of America's dairy land in the 1950s before the interstate highway system was built. Back in those days, cows grazed everywhere in the rolling green fields of Wisconsin. My father had grown up on small farms near Hammond, Wisconsin, during the Depression, helping his parents to raise dairy cattle and other crops during the hardscrabble years before World War II. But for me, my grandparents' farm wasn't the work place my Dad grew up in, but simply the world's best summertime playground.

I remember riding in my Uncle Glenn's old pick-up truck down Wisconsin back roads, singing along to the tinny AM radio, "She wore an itsy-bitsy, teeny-weenie, yellow polka dot bikini ...." *Bikini* was a new word, a French word for a little island in the South Pacific where the mushroom clouds of open air H-Bomb tests billowed up into the atmosphere. My world was fresh, new and simple compared to the tumultuous days of the Roaring Sixties, coming 'round the bend.

In the suburbs of Madison, my brother Bob and I drank milk that came in glass bottles and had cream on the top that we poured over our breakfast cereal. Recalling the fresh, sweet taste, I'm saddened that gradually, over my lifetime, milk products got further and further away from the small family farms of that era, until they became the mass produced products of today. As the years went by, I drank less and less milk, because it didn't seem to have the flavor I remembered when I was young. I also started losing my taste for America's generic cheeses, until I started eating the raw milk and handmade cheeses produced by Europeans, and by small farms in America. They tasted very different!

Milk and Osteoporosis: A Puzzle

Some time before I started writing this book, I began noticing that people I knew were starting to have hip replacement surgery, and that more and more, I was reading in the newspaper about an increase in osteoporosis—all pointing at how us aging baby boomer's bones were somehow deficient. I was puzzled how this could be since Americans consumed more dairy products than anyone in the world. If calcium is good for you, and milk has so much calcium, how come so many Americans have osteoporosis? It just didn't make sense.

When I was a teenager, I traveled in Latin America and was surprised by how healthy people's teeth were in those countries—people who rarely or never drank milk. How could that be, when they didn't consume any dairy? Like most of us in the U.S., I'd been brainwashed into thinking milk was good for you, but I was starting to think maybe it wasn't.

Before I figured out what causes osteoporosis and why some milk is bad and other milk is good—I was very confused. I'd even rejected milk and, like millions of Americans, had started drinking soy milk. I was trying to be health conscious, and I still believed the *unproven theory* that saturated fats and cholesterol are bad for you. So I had quit drinking milk altogether.

Drinking soy milk wasn't much of a replacement, though. I had to admit that soy milk tasted chalky and even beany sometimes. However, *I thought* I was doing my body right by not consuming the BIG BAD CHOLESTEROL and SATURATED FATS in whole milk.

One thing in my favor was I figured out long ago that the only kind of milk to drink is whole milk. I knew this because I once had a co-worker whose family raised hogs in Washington State, and he'd validated my instinctive whole milk bias by telling me how his family raised hogs on skim milk from dairy farms. He only drank whole milk too, and told me how farmers had to pour large quantities of vitamins into the hogs living on *skim* milk, or the hogs would get *scours*, a disease caused by nutritional deficiency. Yet, whole raw milk was excellent for raising hogs and additional vitamins weren't needed.

Occasionally, I run into those who say that milk is designed by nature for baby cows and that humans shouldn't drink it. There's some truth to that, but I think the long and glorious history of producing extremely nutritious, high quality foods from dairy products shows what a one-sided opinion that is. If you want to argue with me about it, I invite you to drink a glass of chalky soy milk and munch on some salty soy nuts while I eat brie cheese on sour dough baguettes and chase it with a glass of chilled, full cream milk from a Guernsey cow. There's good reasons why milk has a long history of human use going back almost 9,000 years!

However, there's many places in the story of milk where I'm going to separate the truth from marketing propaganda, misinformation, disinformation, and ignorance. First of all, modern milk, as sold in America and consumed in enormous quantities, is a seriously defective product that can damage your health. It's a Frankenstein Food that you and your family need to avoid. Industrial milk produced by factory cows and treated and processed in milk and food factories is a far cry from the natural milk produced by grass fed cows living outdoors in the green fields of summer.

Once again, like the cholesterol story, there are two sides to the same coin: there's good milk and there's bad milk. And most of the information you've received all your lifetime has come to you via industry sponsored advertising.

Osteoporosis: The Milk Disease

The best place to start this milk story is by telling you what you need to know about osteoporosis. Then I'll tell you what kind of milk is best to drink to prevent it. We currently have an epidemic of osteoporosis in America, which seems rather strange since we consume so much calcium from dairy products.

Currently, at least five million Americans have been diagnosed with osteoporosis, and over 50 million are judged to be at risk of developing osteoporosis. The current All-American solution to your osteoporosis problem isn't going to the root of the problem and changing your diet, but instead, offers you prescription drugs like Actonel or FosaMax that are only expensive palliatives. Osteoporosis is yet another medical problem in America, where the cure is worse than the problem.

A recent study showed that American women over 50 have some of the highest rates in the world for hip fractures. The only countries with higher rates are Sweden, Finland, Australia and New Zealand. These countries have even higher rates of milk and dairy product consumption than Americans, and consequently, have higher rates of osteoporosis and bone fractures. If milk is so good for you, why do the countries with the highest dairy consumption, have the highest rates of osteoporosis?

Here's the answer you need to know: It's not natural milk that causes osteoporosis—it's the processing of milk that turns it into a defective, dangerous product. From what I learned in writing this chapter, I'll never drink factory milk again.

The best milk to drink is raw, unprocessed, certified milk from healthy cows grazing in green fields or eating organic fodder in the wintertime when green food is unavailable. Seek out raw milk from a dairy farm or small producer near you and pay the extra dollars to get a nutritionally, superior product that's good for you and your family. Drink all you like—the saturated fats and cream in whole milk are the sort of foods your body craves. You'll satisfy your body's natural cravings for fat and be less prone to binge on other foods that aren't good for you.

If you can't get raw milk, you should only drink organic milks—but they're not a perfect food, either. Your average commercial organic whole milk, because of the ultra pasteurization process *might* even have less nutritional value than industrial milk.

If at all possible, you should avoid drinking homogenized milk. I say that with a caveat—drink homogenized milk only if it's the only milk available. There is no proof that milk homogenization is safe. Processing milk by pushing it through tiny stainless steel screens at high pressure and breaking fat globules into very tiny globules, absorbed in a completely different, unnatural way by your body *may* or *may not* be good for you. Drink full cream whole milk that's labeled organic and isn't homogenized and eat cheeses and yoghurts made from raw, unprocessed milk. Nutritionally, these are the best milk foods you can buy.

Drinking milk that isn't pasteurized or homogenized means you are drinking milk as nature intended it to be. Milk is a natural product full of large amounts of calcium, potassium, vitamin C, vitamin D, vitamins and minerals, and live enzymes. Of course, you need to buy milk only from dairy farmers who you know use a high level of cleanliness in producing their fresh milk. The best milk comes from cows that graze on green pastures and have been certified as disease free.

Many states have laws banning the sale of certified raw milk, and agri-business is always trying to do everything possible to prevent your access to the healthiest milk of all. So far, they've also managed to stop the import of the delicious raw cheeses from Europe and have kept the World Trade Organization from allowing these cheeses to be sold in the global market. Hopefully, they'll soon stop their delaying actions, and we'll have some real free trade and can buy high quality, European raw milk cheeses here in America.

LET'S HEAR IT FOR THE SMALL FARMERS IN THE USA!!

We should support small farmers by ending all federal crop support payments to big farmers in America. The perennial problem of American agriculture has always been chronic overproduction. It's a problem a free market place can sort out for itself, without the current system giving large payoffs to America's biggest farmers. Not subsidizing the large farmers (and the clever ones with political connections) is the best way to level the field for the small farmer. There's a bright future for small organic dairy farmers if the government sets standards for selling certified raw milk and allows a natural, healthy product to be sold direct by small farmers to consumers or stores.

Osteoporosis Caused By Magnesium Imbalance

The primary reason why processed dairy products cause osteoporosis is the imbalance of calcium and magnesium. It's not that dairy products are unhealthy. It's a fact that strong and healthy people have used milk for centuries without getting osteoporosis. The problem is the way milk is produced, pasteurized and processed in our modern industrialized countries. The ratio of calcium to magnesium is 10 to 1 in most processed American dairy products. *This is the primary cause of osteoporosis in America,* and I invite you to see my endnotes for this chapter for a host of studies.

Understanding some facts of life about your bones will help you to see what I'm talking about. Bones are living tissues that are constantly being rebuilt. Greatly simplified, there is a two part process that rebuilds your bone tissue. In the first phase, *resorption*, cells called osteoclasts clear old minerals out of bone tissue that has become weak and are carried away in the blood. In the second phase, *mineralization*, osteoblasts deposit new minerals and collagen into areas that have been cleared out. Both osteoblast and osteoclast cells are stimulated by hormones named parathyroid hormone (PTH) and calcitonin (CT). PTH stimulates osteoclasts to pull calcium from the bones, while calcitonin stimulates osteoblasts to deposit calcium in them. When magnesium is lacking, the dynamic balance between PTH and calcitonin tilts toward PTH. This causes excessive stimulation of osteoclasts, which causes net bone loss.

If you consume processed dairy products, taking supplemental magnesium is the *only* way to correct this. If you consume processed dairy products, and you also take calcium tablets—you're doing a serious disservice to your lovely bones.

We know that osteoporosis is lowest in cultures where calcium to magnesium ratios in the diet are 2 to 3, or 3 to 2. Eating large quantities of pasteurized, processed dairy products causes a ratio of total calcium to magnesium in the diet as high as 6 to 1 in Finland and New Zealand. The ratio for the U.S. and Sweden is 5 to 1. No surprise then that all four of these countries have the world's highest consumption of dairy products and the world's highest rates of osteoporosis.

It turns out that African-American women in the U.S. eat over four times as much calcium as African women in Africa, yet they have nine times more osteoporosis. Asian women in the U.S. eat twice the calcium as Asian women in Asia, yet they have three times more osteoporosis. Usually, with increasing affluence, the consumption of dairy products increases and osteoporosis increases. As calcium consumption in Hong Kong and Greece doubled in the last 30 years, the osteoporosis rates tripled in Hong Kong and more than doubled in Greece. Good research shows that the more milk is consumed, the more bone is lost. One of the best studies to prove this—ironically enough, funded by the dairy industry—was published in the *American Journal of Clinical Nutrition* in 1985.

Go Raw and Avoid Osteoporosis

But one thing I wasn't able to find in my research were studies showing calcium and magnesium ratios in raw, unprocessed milks. My guess is those ratios are much better balanced than the ratio in processed milk, or your body absorbs them differently, because of the many enzymes present in a living food. *Pasteurization, of course, kills all natural enzymes in milk.* The test for whether milk has been successfully pasteurized is testing for the presence of enzymes. If they've all been killed off—the milk is pasteurized.

Certified, raw milk builds strong bones and healthy bodies and doesn't cause osteoporosis. It's a product that actually does what milk advertising brags about. Sadly, the industrial milk products sold by America's factory dairies do exactly the opposite. Their products will support life—but you won't have the radiant good health you get from eating living, healthy foods like raw, certified milk.

In China, women get less than 7% of their protein from animal and dairy products and have extremely low levels of osteoporosis. Here in North America, women get 70% of their protein from animal and dairy products and have lots of osteoporosis.

One has to be careful though, extrapolating dietary statistics between different cultures, because there are a lot of other variables. The Chinese eat almost the same amount of eggs and vegetables per capita as Americans, but Americans eat ten times more sugar and six times more fats and oils. Americans eat about 50% more meat and fish per capita, but the Chinese eat almost three times as much grain.

Some scientists and researchers, who have compared the diet of people in China to the American diet and waxed ecstatic about the many benefits of a plant based diet, never mention that the superior health of Chinese peasants might result from other factors in their diet than eating vegetables. Could it be that the benefits came from the low amounts of sugar, white flour, hydrogenated oils, and polyunsaturated oils in the Chinese diet?

I think the statistics on calcium consumption and the tremendous imbalance with magnesium in dairy products are good statistics that clearly point out the problem. The international ratios add credence to the theory that it's the calcium/magnesium imbalance in processed dairy products causing the problem.

If you're going to use processed dairy products, you need to make sure you take magnesium supplements. All the calcium supplements sold are defective products that are poorly absorbed by your body. They only make the calcium/magnesium imbalance worse. Recent studies show inconclusive results as to how much they help prevent osteoporosis. And in one study, the risk of kidney stones among women who took calcium supplements was 17% higher than the control group.

Misleading Marketing

The dairy industry in this country has an enormous amount of marketing clout, and they're always trying to get you to consume more dairy products instead of trying to make a healthier or more nutritious product. Their ads have been misleading and deceptive, to say the least. A recent ad by the California Milk Processors Board in 2005 showed a large picture of a white bone on a black background with the following text:

> *Helmet? Check. Pads? Check. You've seen*
> *what kids try to do on skateboards. They attempt*
> *tricks like sliding down railings. And then try to*
> *land safely on concrete. Maybe that's why broken*
> *forearms are up 42% among kids. On top of that, the*
> *majority of them aren't getting the calcium they need.*
> *So protect your kid on the inside as well as on the*
> *outside. Add some more milk to their diet. Got milk?*

I thought this ad was an interesting spin and a pre-emptive strike on those who might question why the rates of broken forearms are up by 42%. The real question is: Are the increased rates of broken forearms due to sports or from drinking defective, industrial milk products?

Always, the marketing emphasis here in America has been on having lots of calcium in your diet, while magnesium has rarely been mentioned. There should be high levels of magnesium in sea foods, meats, green vegetables and dairy products, but there may not be, due to modern agri-business production methods and milk processing at industrial dairies. We know as many as 80% Americans are magnesium deficient, so this may be why eating seafood as little as twice a week has been shown to cut the risk of heart disease by 30%. Perhaps it's the magnesium that's so lacking in your diet, that getting it from eating seafood is preventing heart attacks. This, of course, is just a supposition—there are a lot of other factors possible in this equation.

Magnesium From Food

I'm going to explain further in this chapter why dairy products are lacking in magnesium, but the lack of magnesium in meats and green vegetables shows you how urgent it is to avoid the industrial foods of American agri-business and eat organic foods. How could it be that magnesium, which makes up as much as 2% of the earth's crust, is missing in action (MIA) in American soils? The reason why Americans are the best fed but malnourished people in the world is that chemical farming processes practiced intensively for over 50 years have bound up naturally occurring minerals in the soil, so plants can't uptake them properly.

One of the easiest ways to make sure you're getting adequate magnesium is to eat homemade broths from chicken, beef or fish. You can also increase your magnesium intake by eating foods such as organic black beans, pinto beans, garbanzo beans, navy beans and squashes which have equal amounts of calcium and magnesium. Also organic spinach, sweet potatoes, green beans, raisins and Brussels sprouts are foods high in both calcium and magnesium. Swiss chard is unusual in that it has almost 50% more magnesium than calcium.

The champion in this department is organic barley which has three times more magnesium than calcium. So, you women who want to have strong and lovely bones wipe off that milk mustache and start eating your barley and Swiss chard....

A History of Milk Corruption

I'm going to continue this story of your daily milk by going back into the history books and telling you how a healthy, natural food like milk got corrupted by politics and whiskey in the aftermath of the war of 1812.

When the War of 1812 with England ended, so did America's supply of hard liquor from the West Indies. The domestic liquor industry started on a large scale, and by 1814, distilleries had sprung up in almost all the major cities of the U.S. As cities expanded, available pasture for cows was reduced, but the demand for corn to make whiskey and milk to feed people increased sharply. Whiskey was, of course, a way to store a perishable crop like corn and add economic value in the process.

The process of fermenting and distilling grains into whiskey left behind an acidic refuse called *distillery slop*. To meet the demand for milk from cows—that no longer grazed so freely—the owners of distilleries began penning up dairy cows next to distilleries and feeding them the hot slop as it came off the stills. This trade came to be known as the *swill milk* or *slop milk* industry.

At first this business developed mostly to get rid of the refuse from distilleries without having to pay to have it hauled away. But when the distillery business contracted in the 1830s, the number of distilleries shrank, and in New York State the number of distilleries dropped to 200. With lower profit margins from whiskey production, more emphasis was put on slop milk production.

Cows feeding on distillery slop yielded an abundance of milk, but that milk was of low quality. Figures from 1852 indicate that in New York City, three quarters of the total milk supply was swill milk. All this milk was produced under abominable conditions and the mortality of dairy animals was incredibly high. The reformer Robert Hartley, an eye witness to the swill dairies, wrote in 1842:

> Here, in a stagnant and empoisoned
> atmosphere that is saturated with the hot steam of
> whiskey slop, and loaded with carbonic acid gas
> and other impurities arising from the excrements of
> hundreds of sickly cattle, they are condemned to live,
> or rather to die on rum-slush. For the space of nine
> months, they are usually tied to the same spot, from
> which, if they live so long, they are not permitted to
> stir, excepting indeed, they become so diseased as to
> be utterly useless for the diary. They are, in a word,
> never unloosed while they are retained as milkers.

By the end of the 19th century, Americans were beginning to realize that the high infant mortalities of almost 50% were connected to the unsanitary milk produced by swill dairies and fed to infants. The poorest people in the country living in urban tenements had the most exposure to dangerous and unhealthy swill milk.

The efforts of reformers such as Robert Hartley educated the public and the next wave of reformers began to change the swill milk situation. In 1889, Henry Coit, M.D., from Newark, New Jersey, started investigating how a system of clean milk production could be started. He formed a committee of 42 physicians whose efforts led to the formation of the first Medical Milk Commission and the beginning of the certified milk movement in America. In 1909, the Medical Milk Commissions Law was passed by both the New Jersey House and Senate. These standards are still used by certified raw milk producers in the states of California, Connecticut, Maine and New Mexico.

More and more milk was being pasteurized at this time, but promoters of certified raw milk saw this as only a stop-gap measure to help public safety until all dairies would produce certified milk on a national level. This was not to be, however, as the methods of another wealthy public-spirited reformer, Nathan Straus, became the most widely used. Nathan Straus promoted pasteurization as the methodology to clean up New York City's milk supply. Straus had made his fortune early in life as a co-owner of Macy's Department Store in New York and dedicated over 30 years of his life advocating for the pasteurization of milk in American and European cities. He had powerful allies, among them Dr. Abraham Jacobi, who served for many years as the head of the American Medical Association.

Nathan Straus was a philanthropist and cleaning up the country's milk supply was his mission. One of his first steps was establishing milk depots where poor people in New York could buy pasteurized milk. Straus sold milk below production cost at his milk depots and by 1916, he had dispensed more than 43 million bottles of pasteurized milk.

Like modern milk today in America, Straus's milk was safe, but of low nutritional quality. Straus was a businessman, and he knew that certified raw milk was expensive to produce, costing two to four times as much as ordinary milk. Pasteurization was a cheap, technological fix for the "milk problem." Because the sloppily produced, contaminated raw milk of the 1880s caused so much disease and death among young children, pasteurization was welcomed; it made milk safer and was a cheap source of food for poor people.

From the beginning, the proponents of pasteurization failed to realize it wasn't the nature of milk itself, but the way it was produced that made the milk unhealthy. They failed to realize that pasteurizing milk destroys much of milk's nutritional value.

Pasteurization found an important ally when Straus got President Teddy Roosevelt to conduct a study of the milk problem in 1907. A committee of 20 government experts stated that pasteurization doesn't change the chemical composition, taste, digestibility or nutritive qualities of milk. These "facts" are still repeated today and persist in official government literature, despite overwhelming evidence to the contrary. As early as 1912, influential and powerful voices in government were already urging compulsory pasteurization of all milk produced in America, even certified milk. Businessmen were starting to invest large sums of capital building pasteurization plants, and the public health and medical authorities were on board for requiring mandatory pasteurization of all milk.

A short term gain for public health by cleaning up the swill dairies turned into a long term loss for the public health, once mandatory pasteurization became accepted. *Pasteurization and ultra pasteurization destroy much of milk's quality as a food, and it's a loss for our health having such a healthy, natural food as raw milk degraded.*

The enzymes that are destroyed when milk is pasteurized are *galactase, peroxidase, catalase, amylase, lipase, lactase,* and *phosphatase.* The heat treatment also alters the amino acids *lysine* and *tyrosine,* and makes unsaturated fats go rancid quicker. Vitamin C content is reduced anywhere between 10 to 50%, and smaller amounts of vitamins B6 and B12 are destroyed. Some advocates of raw milk have stated that more vitamin C is destroying in pasteurizing milk than is contained in the entire U.S. citrus crop. Cheap synthetic D vitamins are added, and chemicals are often added to enhance taste and suppress odors.

Pasteurization also alters and affects the availability of the mineral components of milk, such as calcium, chloride, phosphorus, magnesium, sodium, potassium, sulphur and many trace minerals. Powdered skim milk, produced by commercial dehydration that oxidizes the cholesterol and makes it harmful to your arteries, is added to most milk. This ultra high temperature drying process also creates free *glutamic acid* that is toxic to the central nervous system, and cross-linked proteins and nitrate compounds that are known carcinogenic compounds. You won't see powdered skim milk on the label though, because its addition is regarded as an "industry standard practice," and disclosure isn't required.

When high standards of cleanliness aren't required in the production of milk, producers often rely upon the pasteurization process to deal with fecal matter, dirt and bacteria in milk. Most industrial milk is pasteurized as many as three times to deal with this problem. Contrary to popular belief, pasteurization does not give complete guarantees of safety, as recent outbreaks of *salmonella* and *listeria* have occurred in pasteurized milk. Interestingly enough, raw milk contains strains of lactic acid producing bacteria that protect against pathogens. However, pasteurization destroys these helpful bacteria designed by nature to protect against inadvertent contamination. These bacteria are the reason raw milk slowly turns sour, instead of putrefying like pasteurized milk. If strict procedures for producing certified milk are adhered to, the same technologies of milking machines, stainless steel tanks, and quick chilling are the ones that make pasteurization *unnecessary*.

Some Other Problems of Industrial Milk

Besides the enormous problems with the imbalances of calcium and magnesium and the loss of so many nutrients, some of the other big problems are the growth hormones, antibiotics, and pesticide residues you ingest when you drink pasteurized and homogenized industrial milk. Growth hormones are used to stimulate greater milk production, but end up producing a lower quality of milk.

A little known problem is the dilution of vitamins in industrial milk. Dairy cows that graze in the traditional manner on grass fields usually produce two or three gallons of high quality natural milk daily. In contrast, some of today's Holstein cows raised in factory farms produce over eight gallons daily. Of course, the vitamins are diluted in milk produced in such copious quantities.

This abnormally high milk production is accomplished by selective breeding of cows with overactive pituitary glands, using high protein feeds, and injecting cows with a product named Posilac from Monsanto Corporation. Posilac is widely known as the bovine growth hormone, *rBGH*.

Cows with overactive pituitary glands already produce milk with large amounts of *insulin-like growth factor* (IGF-I), which is a perfect match between humans and cows. IGF-I is the most powerful growth hormone in the human body, and every sip of milk and every bite of cheese contains IGF-I. The huge consumption of dairy products in America and ingestion of excess amounts of bovine growth hormones *may* be the prime reason why menstruation occurs at ages 11 and 12 in young women in America versus age 16 or 17 in China.

Monsanto's marketing of the genetically engineered, synthetic growth hormone rBGH, now used by over one third of the dairy herds in the U.S., supercharges the levels of IGF-I (growth hormone) to even higher levels. These levels are increased further when milk is pasteurized. The purpose of rBGH is to increase milk production, and injecting this hormone does exactly that—milk production increases by over 10%. Why this is desirable when America is always dealing with chronic milk overproduction, is rather puzzling.

ONLY DRINK MILK THAT SAYS NO RBGH ON THE LABEL OR DRINK MILK PRODUCED BY LOCAL FARMERS
Here are the real facts:
rBGH makes cows ill. Monsanto has had to admit to almost 20 toxic effects, including mastitis, on the drug label for Posilac.
rBGH milk is chemically and nutritionally different from natural milk.
rBGH milk is often contaminated with pus from mastitis induced by using rBGH. It also often contains antibiotics used to treat mastitis.
The high levels of IGH-I have been well documented for causing breast cancers, prostate and colon cancers.
Some industry studies show that rBGH milk may have levels of IGF-I as much as 10 times higher than normal.
IGF-I blocks natural defense mechanisms known as *apoptosis* that work against early growth of submicroscopic cancers.

Based upon strong scientific evidence, Canada, Norway, Switzerland, New Zealand, Japan, and 28 nations of the European Union have all banned the use and import of rBGH tainted milk products from the U.S. The Food and Drug Administration is still ignoring these problems and strongly supports Monsanto's position on rBGH. Monsanto has powerful influence because of its many interlocking connections with the American Medical Association, The American Cancer Society, and the Republican Party that has ruled Washington most of the last 20 years.

One of the strongest voices to speak up against Monsanto was Congressman John Conyers, Chair of the House Committee on Government Operations. I found the following quote by him mentioned in a citizen's petition to the FDA to take Monsanto's bovine growth hormone off the market posted on the website of the Organic Consumers Association: "I find it reprehensible that Monsanto and the FDA have chosen to suppress and manipulate animal health test data in efforts to approve commercial use of rBGH…without regard to the adverse effects on humans."

Got Organic?

I thought I was doing my body a world of good by giving up soy milk and going back to drinking whole, organic milk, but once I knew more about milk, I realized again, I was making a mistake. I hope I can help you decipher this modern world we live in as I stumble along this pilgrim's path.

I soon realized that the organic milk I started to drink was produced by Horizon Corporation, and it turns out they control over 50% of the organic milk market in the U.S. I thought I was buying milk from cows raised on grass, as their advertising labels suggest, but that wasn't what I was getting. Horizon's cows eat organic grain and hay, but their cows are heavy producers contained in fenced dry lots, mostly in Western states, on gigantic milk production facilities. It's a long way from milk produced by cows grazing on green grass in the fields of Wisconsin. Ahhh, Progress—Ain't it Grand?

And the other surprise was that most of the milk from Horizon and another organic producer, Organic Cow of Vermont, turned out to be ultra pasteurized milk. In conventional pasteurization, milk is heated to 145 degrees for 30 minutes. Ultra pasteurization, also known as UHT (ultra high temperature), heats milk to 285 degrees, way above the boiling point of 212. All the microorganisms that might spoil the milk are killed and the milk is aseptically packaged. These milk products can be stored unopened at room temperature up to six months. They're sold in the refrigerator section though, because American consumers would be unlikely to purchase milk if they thought it didn't need refrigeration.

Organic milk commands a premium in the grocery store, yet it *might* be substantially less nutritious than regular, pasteurized milk. Wouldn't it be nice, if the FDA weren't a highly politicized organization, and could actually check out a situation like this and let you know what the truth is?

The Diseased State of Today's Milk

The changes in milk production have been enormous in my short lifetime. In 1950, there were 5.4 million farms and 3.7 million of them had dairy cows. Almost all of them were raised on grass in pastures. By the year 2000, there were less than 2 million farms and only 102,250 of them had milk cows. In the year 2000, America passed another futuristic goal—over 50% of the milk was produced on farms with more than 500 cows.

Almost all of today's dairy cows are being raised under the "grim, steel roofs" of confinement facilities and never get to graze on green grass. The average lifespan for a containment facility dairy cow is 42 months compared to a lifespan of 12 to 15 years for a dairy cow living in green pastures. A common food now used for high milk production is high protein fodder, such as soybean meal. This fodder generates high milk production but leads to sterility, liver problems, shortened lives, and high rates of *mastitis*, or infected mammary glands.

Very little research has been done on how these foods alter the nutritional profile of milk from that of cows feeding on green grass. It's also possible the high rate of milk allergies in infants and young children could be correlated to dairy cattle being fed such unnatural fodder. This high protein feed also causes stomach problems in dairy cows that often require the use of large amounts of antibiotics.

According to the National Mastitis Council, nearly 40% of all dairy cattle have some form of mastitis. When cows' mammary glands are infected, there are large amounts of pus excreted along with the milk. Rather shocking, isn't it, to think that 40% of the milk you drink *might* contain large amounts of pus and antibiotics? This is why they pasteurize milk more than once—heat is used to neutralize the pus and bacteria in the milk. Ultra pasteurization is also used to gloss over this problem—as Monsanto, the FDA, and the National Mastitis Council might say—that pus and bacteria in your milk is perfectly sterile.

Obviously, when you zip into 7/11 and buy a gallon of milk for $2, there's a price to be paid. What did you expect—the green pastures, the sun, the moon, the stars, and free crème brulee and crème fraiche too? If you care about your health, you need to buy high quality dairy foods from farmers who produce natural, healthy products.

I'd be remiss if I didn't take the time to mention the possible connection with Crohn's disease and Johne's (pronounced yo-neez) disease. Johne's disease is a common ailment of cattle with symptoms of chronic or intermittent diarrhea, emaciation and death. The contagious organism that causes the disease, *Mycobacterium avium paratuberculosis* (Map), lives in the intestines, proliferates in the udder, and is excreted into the milk of infected cows. About 40 % of the dairy herds in the US are infected and the numbers are increasing.

The modern containment facilities for industrial milk production are an optimum environment for the spread of a disease such as the Map bacterium. This is because the Map bacterium is hard to detect and culture, and only a small percentage of infected cows with no microscopically visible organisms will test positive. In humans, the microbe also often goes undetected because it's hard to detect using standard lab procedures. Few people in the general public have heard of Johne's disease, but it's a topic of great concern in the dairy industry, one they'd very much like to keep out of the public eye.

The diary industry has been slow in admitting possible relationships between Johne's disease in cattle and Crohn's disease in humans. Most of the medical researchers studying Crohn's disease believe it's an autoimmune disease. A core group of researchers continue studies finding disturbing links between Johne's disease and Crohn's disease.

One of the leading experts on Crohn's disease is Dr. George Herman-Taylor, the head of surgery at St. George's Medical School in London. He was quoted in 2002 in the *Wisconsin Agriculturist*, saying, "When the evidence is considered, it's difficult to argue the case that the organism is not involved. It is certain that M. paratuberculosis can be pathogenic in humans and that it's very likely that it causes a significant proportion—even a substantial proportion—of Crohn's disease in humans."

Both dairy industry spokesmen and the FDA state that pasteurization is the only way to kill pathogenic organisms in milk, but the problem in this situation is that the Map bacterium causing Johne's disease *survives* pasteurization. Testing in New England between 1990 and 1995 showed the Map bacterium was present in 7% of all milk samples tested, and the probability these organisms had survived pasteurization was high. Many of those afflicted with Crohn's disease are becoming angry with the dairy industry and their perceived lack of interest in investigating the links between Johne's disease and Crohn's disease.

If you are diagnosed with Crohn's disease, like a few young people recently have in Santa Barbara, you will be told it's an incurable disease, your prognosis is bad, and you will be facing a lifetime of doctor visits, steroid use, and possible abdominal surgeries. The medical journals call this new disease an autoimmune disorder involving the small intestine that causes malabsorption and inhibits maturation and growth. It's a new disease—and a bad one for young people.

Some of those in Santa Barbara with this disease have put it into full remission by not eating sugar, grains, soy and wheat, and by taking nutritional supplements and pro-biotic acidophilus bacteria. The dietary regimen is made up of a nutrient dense variety of vegetables, fruits, legumes, ground nuts, and proteins. I'll include some recipes in the last chapter, suitable for those suffering from Crohn's disease.

The dairy industry's response to Johne's disease is to reluctantly move towards testing and to attempt to develop new pharmaceuticals to combat Johne's disease. Also, the higher temperatures of ultra pasteurization are thought by many in the industry to be the solution to the problem. A much simpler solution is to return our country's dairy animals to green pastures and to drink raw certified milk. The beneficial bacteria in raw milk are supremely well adapted to deal with pathogens such as the Map bacterium. And because raw milk is so much easier to digest and provides superior nourishment, it doesn't provide a beneficial environment in your gut for the Map bug, as industrial milk does.

Full Circle Swill

I'm going to end this chapter of milk by telling you how we've come full circle from the swill milk era of the late 1890s all the way to our current era when dairy cattle are fed on "distiller's grain," a byproduct of ethanol production at industrial milk factories. Hold your nose—this story, reported in the *Wall Street Journal* in 2006, isn't quite what you had in mind when you thought of recycling. This time, the economies of scale in American business have led us all the way to Hereford, Texas, and the mountains of bullshit piled up as far as the eye can see around this not-so-scenic Texas town. Stink? You think? *No, mah friend and fellah American—that's the smell of money in Hereford, Texas.*

It's interesting how the slop of whiskey distilleries fed to captive dairy cows in the late 1800s has appeared again in our modern day of industrial milk. Milk is once again being produced from cows being fed on residue from distilleries. Only this time, giant industrial plants in Hereford are busy cooking the corn grown in America's heartland down to alcohol to fuel automobiles, not whiskey.

Of course, all this ethanol is being grown with enormous crop and cash subsidies from Uncle Sugar in Washington, D.C., or this screwy process wouldn't be happening. The only "green" re-cycling being done is the political influence peddling done through federal crop subsidies paid out to corporate farmers. Most of the crop subsidies paid out to big corporate farmers gets cashed in Midwest states, which are critical states for electoral votes. Iowa is, of course, Ground Zero for presidential primaries. To keep the best possible cash flow coming to America's corporate farmers, crop subsidies are paid to guarantee prices—or they can get paid for not growing crops. Only the tax payer (America's sucker of last resort) could think something might be wrong with this scheme.

I respect my fellow Americans who want to go green, but the primary reason the ethanol business is booming is because of crop support prices paid to corn growers and the generous subsidies and tax incentives for ethanol producers. The petroleum energy input into growing and producing corn is about equal to the energy gained from making ethanol fuel out of corn. The question is: Does Zero equal Zero in Washington, D.C.? This ethanol fuel program has worked in

Brazil, because it's at least three times more efficient making ethanol from sugar cane than corn. This entire program of ethanol production has little to do with energy independence and much to do with political corruption in Washington, D.C.

But back to our story about the symbiotic relationships between the feedlots, ethanol plants, and dairy cows in good old Hereford, Texas. This is a town that's had a serious manure problem for a long time. The stuff keeps piling up around the enormous feedlots around the town. The one million cattle on the town's feedlots are a $2.7 billion annual business, but the town has always had to deal with the 6,300 tons of manure they generate every day.

Don't forget that livestock production in the U.S. produces about 130 times as much manure as humans. The folks in Hereford have tried burning it to generate electricity, shipping it away for fertilizer and making pellets for wood stoves, but now they're finally starting to get a leg up on their manure problem. The ethanol plants are burning manure as a fuel source and cooking corn into ethanol. Then they feed the left over by-products of distiller's grain back to feed lot cattle and dairy cows. Viola! Re-cycling, Texas style!

Recently, Hereford has persuaded (with cash and tax breaks) 10 dairies from Texas, California, Idaho, Texas, and New Mexico to relocate more than 60,000 of their cows to containment facilities in Hereford, Texas. Dairy cows eat more than feed lot cattle, so they often produce as much as four times more manure. As Todd Carter, the President of Panda Energy and builder of the newest and largest ethanol plant said in the *Wall Street Journal*, "We're taking the manure from one end, and then feeding them the distiller's grain. So there are certain synergies."

I'll Take It Raw

I don't know about you, but my choice of synergies is the natural alchemy that occurs between the sun making green grass and healthy cows eating it, and making certified whole raw milk that I can buy from my local farmer in a glass bottle. And the next phase of the alchemy is for someone to make natural, healthy milk into fine butter, cream, and cheeses.

The best thing I suggest you do for your health and your family's good health is to consume less industrial milk, and find a place to buy certified raw milk from a local farmer near you. Always try and buy dairy products made from milk that isn't pasteurized or homogenized. Help America's small organic dairy farmers by buying the healthy and nutritious products they produce with pride right here in America.

CHAPTER SEVEN

The Great Soy Menace To Your Health

Soy food products have become big business in America. Like many Americans, you may have started eating products made from these high protein beans–tofu, soy milk, veggie burgers—as a substitute for the high-cholesterol foods we've been warned are harmful. The truth about soy foods is very different: most soy foods are a serious hazard to your good health.

Soy Enlightenment

When I first started my research for this book, I thought, like most people, I should be careful not to eat too much red meat, seafood, milk, butter or eggs, because those foods contained cholesterol. At that time, I still believed the dominant paradigm that eating too much cholesterol was unhealthy. This, is of course, the official opinion of the American Heart Association and the American Medical Association.

As I started cutting back on cholesterol and trying to figure out the best possible diet, I gave up eating butter, milk, and meat as much as possible. I did this because like most of you, I trusted the consensus opinions of medical experts and researchers. Being over 50, I wanted to be healthy, so I started drinking soy milk, ate more vegetables and grains, drank fruit smoothies with silken tofu, cut back on red meat and seafood, and started finding ways to eat tofu as a main course.

I soon realized this diet program made me feel tired a lot of the time. I felt as tired as if I'd gone to the other extreme and overindulged in rich, fatty foods. Also, eating this way made me start to crave fats. If you've ever tried to live on an ultra-low saturated fats diet, loaded with vegetable protein, you understand these cravings. Eat this diet for too long, and unless you're a Buddhist monk—you'll want pizza, a hamburger and a milkshake delivered to your house, ASAP!

By experimenting with my diet and cutting down drastically on saturated fats and cholesterol, I soon realized that the diet our medical authorities in America recommend, not only doesn't make you feel good—it's almost impossible to stay on it. It's just not natural—your body doesn't like it. I found out that most of the diet plans marketed in my lifetime and recommendations made by "experts" didn't pan out too well. I studied all of the dietary programs I could find, from Zen macrobiotic diets, to Atkins, to the South Beach Diet to Dr. Phil's Diet Plan, and couldn't find any that made sense. There are good reasons why you can buy copies of most of these books at your local used book store.

One of the most extreme diets I researched was the Pritikin Plan, as recommended by Nathaniel Pritikin. It was a low protein, low fat and high carbohydrate diet that didn't allow you to eat any butter, oils, or red meats. Pritikin's opinion was that supplements weren't necessary and foods should provide all your vitamins and minerals. All foods—vegetables and meats—had to be either steamed or boiled. On the positive side, he recommended eating no sugar, white flour, or processed foods. He also advocated eating healthy raw foods and doing vigorous work outs.

This was a popular diet, but few people had the willpower to stay on such a strict regimen for long. You find yourself having low energy levels, being mildly depressed, having trouble concentrating, and eventually being deficient in minerals and vitamins. Nathaniel Pritikin realized this diet wasn't working and modified it by adding some fat to the diet. Sadly, he suffered from depression—partly from eating a diet like this—and probably from realizing his diet program wasn't working. He avoided heart disease but eventually was diagnosed with leukemia, and in the prime of life, committed suicide.

Perhaps you might feel depressed, too, if you've ever been dedicated enough to stay on a severe dietary regimen for long. I wasn't feeling too good myself, as I realized my diet full of tofu, soy milk, and vegetables wasn't such a good idea. I kept trying to eat more and more tofu by finding ways to flavor it and eat it as a main course.

As I continued in my research for this book, still sticking to a soy-dominant diet, I discovered some of the new health books that thoroughly debunked the idea cholesterol is bad for you. As I mentioned in Chapter Two, probably the best book is by Swedish doctor Uffe Ravnskov, *The Cholesterol Myths, Exposing the Fallacy that Saturated Fats and Cholesterol Cause Heart Disease*. Many of you reading this book may still accept the failed theory that natural cholesterol in your diet is dangerous. Or perhaps, the points I raised in earlier chapters have provoked you to think about it—but you're not completely convinced just yet.

Once you realize high quality cholesterol is good for you, then you have to ask the question: *Why on earth would anyone drink soy milk on a regular basis or try to live on tofu or garden burgers?* Its a noble thing to live your life with the Buddhist and Hindu concepts of not killing animals to eat them, but when it comes to nutrition, if you don't eat fish, meat, milk, cheese, or even eggs, you would have to put a great deal of effort into making sure you're eating a nutritionally sound diet.

If you eat soy foods as part of your vegetarian diet, you may think you're doing a good thing. But to benefit from soy foods, you need to consume soy foods in the traditional forms—tempeh, tofu, miso, and natto—and only as they've been made for centuries in Asia, not their processed forms as manufactured by American agri-business companies, such as Con-Agra, Monsanto, Dean Foods, Kraft, Heinz and Cargill. Despite their advertising claims, these companies' concern is not your health, but the profits of their shareholders. Much of the newest marketing of soybeans has been aimed at intelligent, educated consumers who are being led to believe soy is a "green," environmentally safe, and healthful alternative to meat production. The truth is very different. Many soy products are a serious health hazard and a menace to your well being.

Around the same time I discovered that cholesterol is good for you and that a low fat lifestyle is bad for your health, I started reading Kaayla T. Daniel's landmark book, *The Whole Soy Story*. If you're a vegetarian, a vegan, or anyone who's ever tried to consume large quantities of soy, you need to get a copy of her book and study it thoroughly. She's a nutritional pioneer and the first to publish a mainstream, mass market book telling of the many dangers of soy products. If you're interested in healthy living, her book is as important as *Silent Spring* was in its day.

Kaayla is a big wave surfer, riding a groundswell of interest in healthy living and good nutrition, and I can't praise her book enough. Like her, I'm hoping I can change the dietary habits of mainstream Americans so we can all live long, productive and healthy lives. The tremendous amount of dietary misinformation has now created a general populace so unhealthy that Americans spend over $6,000 per capita on medical care, and we're some of the unhealthiest people in the world.

The Soy Food Menace

One of the primary reasons why Americans are so sick is because of the mass consumption of foods and oils produced from soybeans. In researching this book, nothing could have surprised me more than discovering how so many products manufactured from soybeans and sold as heart-healthy, low fat and low cholesterol, are actually a menace to your health. Vegetarians and vegans in particular are also being duped by slick advertising for soy foods that are as dangerous as the mainstream, low fat convenience foods sold in supermarkets and the high fat foods eaten by fast food customers. All of these "foods" contain dangerous amounts of soybean products deleterious for your health. The common thread in all three diets—the vegetarian diet, the low fat food diet and the high fat junk food diet—is the unnatural, manufactured soy foods they contain. It really is this simple: *Soy beans are not a health food.*

Modern American agricultural businesses are currently marketing soybean products and oils all over the world as a natural, healthy, low-calorie, anti-cancer food rich in vital nutrients and good for your heart and for balancing your hormones. Nothing could be further from the truth. American agri-business chooses to ignore what the Chinese and the Japanese learned long ago—that soybeans must be soaked, cooked, and fermented in order to transform them into healthy food. This is because soybeans naturally contain large amounts of anti-nutrients, such as *trypsin* inhibitors, *saponins*, *lectins*, and *phytates* that are growth suppressing factors.

Modern processing methods deal with this "soybean nutrition problem" by treatment with high heat and with oxidizers, such as hydrogen peroxide, acids, and solvents, such as hexane, to improve the flavor and texture. Other chemicals and solvents are used to de-activate phytates and other anti-nutrient factors in soybeans. Without such processing, soy protein is difficult to digest, causes flatulence, is nutritionally deficient, and is full of plant hormones that interfere with your body's regulation of testosterone or estrogen.

Only traditional Asian methods of processing, as distinct from modern chemical processing, can transform soybeans into healthy food. Asian societies have never eaten soybean products in quantity or as main courses. Soy milk also was never consumed in quantity in any traditional Asian society. It's a chalky tasting, nutritionally deficient product that makes as much sense to drink as milk made from left-over margarine.

In health books such as *The Okinawa Diet* and *Diet for a New America*, authors have maintained that Asian societies derive health benefits from high usage of soy products. But in Okinawa, the actual foods consumed by some of the healthiest people in the world turned out to be very different than how they were represented by health book authors. Surprisingly enough, the most common cooking oil on Okinawa is not soy oil or canola oil, but good old fashioned fat from pigs—that's right, *lard,* according to genontologist Kazuhhiko Taira. Another surprise is that healthy Okinawans eat about four ounces each day of both pork and fish. They eat a lot of vegetables and small amounts of soy products. And all of the soy products they consume (miso, tofu, and soy sauce) are traditional fermented or precipitated soy foods.

The many advocates of soy foods commonly make the claim that soy is a staple food in Asian societies. The truth is that the people of Korea, Mongolia, Vietnam, Thailand, Indonesia, China and even Japan don't eat very much soy. As recently as 1977, a publication, *Food in Chinese Culture,* stated that soy foods account for 1.5% of calories in the Chinese diet versus 65% of calories from pork.

The Story of Soy in America and the World

The soy story in America starts with the soybean's historical use as a nitrogen fixing cover crop. The closest relatives to soybean are clover, peas, and alfalfa, which all have the capability to take nitrogen from the atmosphere and fix it in the soil. Unlike other plants that take nitrogen from the soil or water, the soybean's capability to fix nitrogen in the soil makes it extremely valuable in American agriculture.

Today, growing and processing soybeans has become the cornerstone of America's manufactured food industry. Almost all processed foods today contain varying amounts of soy oil, soy flour, soy protein isolates, and textured soy proteins. The demonization of saturated fats and cholesterol in natural healthy foods, such as meat, milk, cheese, cream, eggs, and butter has been an incredible boon to the soy industry.

As recently as the 1950s, the soybean industry had a tremendous disposal problem with the left over sludge from manufacturing soy oils and margarine. For many years, these by-products were used for livestock and poultry food, fish farms, and fertilizers, but now, due to modern processing, they're blended into thousands of processed foods. Due to the ingenuity of American food processors and manufacturers, what used to be fish or chicken feed is now packaged and sold as veggie burgers, tofu sausage, Tofutti ice cream, or chocolate soy milk.

Annually, well over $100 million is spent marketing soybeans in America. Other countries have followed our lead and jumped into farming soybeans on a large scale. In South America, rain forest and virgin lands are being converted into soybean production by agribusiness at an ever increasing pace. Because of global competition, America's share of soybean production has declined from over 50% down to about 35%. Brazil currently produces about 30%, Argentina produces 17% and China produces about 8%. China currently imports more soybeans than they produce.

A shocking fact, not well known, is that as much as two-thirds of the soybeans grown in the U.S. are genetically modified (GM) soybeans patented and marketed by the Monsanto Corporation. Monsanto spent millions of dollars and many years before succeeding in developing a genetically modified strain of soybeans that were resistant to Monsanto's highly profitable weed killer, Roundup. It wasn't until Monsanto scientists were able to genetically splice a hardy bacterium discovered in sewage at a Monsanto plant into a patented soybean plant, that they achieved their goal.

Monsanto's genetically modified soybean plants were rushed to market in 1996, and their FDA approval was obtained on the basis there was little difference between genetically modified soybeans and conventional beans. But many scientists who have looked at Monsanto's testing methods of their new soybean feel the tests were incomplete and rigged to reach a favorable conclusion for their new product launch.

Among the many concerns of scientists not on Monsanto's payroll, are elevated hormone levels in genetically modified beans, lower protein levels, low levels of the essential amino acid *phenylalanine*, lowered body weights of male test rats, and adverse effects to the kidneys, liver and testicles of male test rats. Accusations of false summation of the data, protocols designed to produce predetermined results, misinterpretation of data, and selective citation have led to demands for independent scientific tests to determine the safety of Monsanto's patented, genetically modified soybeans.

At the present time, I repeat for emphasis, these new genetically modified beans comprise *two-thirds* of the soybeans grown in the U.S. Are they safe? Unless the Food and Drug administration starts doing the job it's supposed to do, how will we ever know?

Before Monsanto, and outside of the U.S., some of the more avid promoters of soy foods are a rogue's gallery, including the vegetarian Adolph Hitler, Italian dictator Benito Mussolini, Cuban president Fidel Castro, and the government of the USSR. A little history: In 1929, Benito Mussolini ordered the formation of the Committee for the Study of Soya to help expand the use of soy flours in Italian foods. In Cuba in 1995, the persistent shortage of dairy products led the Cuban government to distribute free soy milk and soy yoghurt to children between ages 7 and 14. Fidel Castro, history's most successful revolutionary, had to use soybeans to make faux milk to take the heat off his singular mis-management of Cuba's economy. And in the '50s and '60s, the Communist Party in the USSR pushed for expanded production of soy margarine and soy proteins as an inexpensive solution to Russia's chronic food production problems under communist governance.

Food manufacturers here in North America currently use soy beans as a feed stock to make thousands of food products. One of the most ubiquitous "soy foods" is called *soy protein isolate*, or SPI. SPI is added to almost everything from hamburgers to bread. Surprisingly enough, the soy protein isolate currently added to thousands of manufactured foods in America has never received certification as a GRAS (Generally Recognized As Safe) additive to food by the FDA.

In 1979, the Select Committee of GRAS Substances (SCOGS) looked at public safety issues in manufacturing soy protein isolates. The Committee advised establishing acceptable levels of carcinogenic *nitrosamines* and *nitrites*, and monitoring the toxic amino acid *lysinoalanine* in edible food products. To date, this has not been done by the FDA, and currently, soy protein isolates are even added to baby formula. The amount the SCOGS committee recommended in 1979 for maximum safe exposure to soy protein isolates was 150 milligrams. Americans now eat over ten times as much soy protein isolates as they did in 1979, and vegetarians might consume as much as 100 times more than the amount considered safe by the SCOG committee in 1979.

Surprisingly enough, soy protein isolates were not initially developed as a food product. In the late 1970s, the Federation of American Society for Experimental Biology (FASEB) decided that a safe use for soy protein isolates was as a sealer for cardboard boxes. However, they expressed concern over the potential for carcinogenic nitrosamines and the toxic amino acid lysinoalanine leaching from the soy protein isolate used as a sealer into the contents of the cardboard boxes. Clearly, it would have been unimaginable to the Committee that soy protein isolate would eventually be packaged in cardboard boxes and sold as a product—and with claims made on the side of the box that it was good for your health. How things have changed since 1979.

Soy and Your Heart

As mentioned in Chapter Five, with the approval of aspartame (Thank you, Donald Rumsfield!) and the marketing of Splenda, ever since the Reagan Revolution took over Washington in 1980, your government has been for sale to the highest bidder. Science has been kicked out the door and sent packing, and the FDA has been emasculated by politicians who have delivered the goods to Big Pharma, food processors and American agri-business. If you're an American, you live in a country where industries have been allowed to regulate themselves, and they've done so to benefit their shareholders—not the health of you and your family. When it comes to food, both Republicans and Democrats have handed over the keys of the chicken coop to the world's corporate foxes.

In October of 1999, the FDA approved the health claim prominently displayed on soy products that reads: "According to the FDA, 25 grams of soy protein a day, when consumed as part of a diet low in saturated fat and cholesterol, may reduce the risk of heart disease." This health claim approved by the FDA is what made soy sales soar in the last ten years.

The story of how this claim was certified by the FDA is about as fraudulent as the approval of aspartame as a sugar substitute. The original petition was submitted to the FDA by Protein Technologies International, requesting the health claim, not for soy protein but for *soy isoflavones,* the plant-based estrogens found in abundance in soybeans. Given the evidence was weak that isoflavones lower cholesterol, and the evidence was strong of their toxicity and endocrine system disruption, the FDA should have been duty bound to throw out the petition. But they didn't. Violating their own rules of only ruling on substances presented by petition, the FDA took the unprecedented step of throwing out Protein Technologies International's petition and substituting a claim for *soy protein* instead of the one for *soy isoflavones.* Further stacking the deck, the FDA shortened the approval process by limiting the time to 30 days in which members of the public could comment or protest the proposed ruling.

In order to allow this health claim and benefit soybean producers and manufacturers, the FDA disregarded the testimony of scientists at the FDA's National Center for Toxological Research, British researchers, and other experts who provided evidence of possible danger from the biologically active *isoflavones, phytates* and *goitrogens* (substances blocking the synthesis of thyroid hormones), and allergens in soy beans. These concerns were dismissed in favor of weak evidence that soy might lower cholesterol and to support the widely believed—yet never proven—theory that cholesterol lowering is important in preventing cardio-vascular disease.

To approve this health claim for soy, the FDA relied almost entirely on a 1995 meta-analysis by James W. Anderson, PhD. The trend to use meta-analyses of studies is an increasing trend among researchers and their sponsors in industry. Many scientists have criticized the authors of meta-analyses for using them to support flawed assumptions or for deleting scientific studies that contradict desired conclusions. Anderson deleted eight studies that didn't support the desired conclusion, and he included 29 studies that offered some proof that replacing animal protein with soy protein would bring about a 7 to 20% lowering of cholesterol levels in individuals with cholesterol levels of 260 mg/dl or higher. However, for individuals with cholesterol levels of 250 mg/dl or less, the studies showed soy protein is unlikely to lower cholesterol levels and might even slightly raise them. Even worse, for the majority of people who might consume 25 grams or more of soy protein, there's lots of scientific evidence pointing at serious disruption of your endocrine system and possible damage to your thyroid gland.

The best possible evidence demonstrated by this fraudulent health claim on soy products is that the FDA is not only asleep at the wheel, but has jumped into bed with the very people they're supposed to be regulating.

Soy Isoflavones — Cure for Cancer?

If bogus health claims to prevent osteoporosis and heart disease weren't enough for you to stomach, the soy industry is now attempting to sell you soy proteins and soy isoflavones as a cure for cancer. In 2004, the Solae Company petitioned the FDA for the right to make a cancer health claim for soy proteins. As reported in *The Whole Soy Story*, Solae stated in their petition: "There is scientific agreement among experts qualified by scientific training and experience to evaluate such claims regarding the relationship between soy protein products and a reduced risk of certain cancers."

The preposterous idea that scientists (at least those not on the soy industry's payroll!) would consider soy products for an anti-cancer claim is laughable. *Soy isoflavones*—soybean estrogens often marketed as preventing cancer—are listed as carcinogens in the American Chemical Society's 1976 chemical carcinogens list. One of the front men in the advertising blitz for soy isoflavones as a cure for cancer is former Junk Bond King, Michael Milliken. It's a made-in-America soap opera—the Michael Milliken Story—someone who was banned from Wall Street for life, fresh out of prison, recovered from prostate cancer—and now selling you questionable cancer cures made from soybeans!

One of the marketing pitches for these soy "medicines" is that the rate from breast cancer is four times lower in China than in the U.S., and the rate of prostate cancer is 18 times lower. The good health of people in China is being attributed to their high consumption of soy foods by soybean promoters here in America. The facts however don't back the media hype of anti-cancer soy marketers. As I mentioned earlier—the Chinese don't eat very much soy. And if the decreased rates of breast and prostrate cancer are attributed to soy consumption, then it would be logical for soy to take the blame for the increased rates of liver, pancreas, stomach, and thyroid cancers in Asia. Many studies show reduced incidents of cancer with soy use, but they also show reductions correlated with rice, green tea, fruits, fish and vegetables. Those who examine the many laboratory studies on anti-cancer effects of soy can only state that the results are contradictory.

More likely, the scientific explanation of the substantially lower rates of breast and prostrate cancer in China is their lack of exposure to synthetic hormones in plastics, agricultural pesticides, and synthetic growth hormones and chemicals used in raising industrial pork, chicken, and beef here in the U.S. Americans also consume more chemicals and toxins because they eat 50% more meat and fish per capita than the Chinese do. Another possibility is that the Chinese have much healthier immune systems because they only eat 10% as much sugar and 15% as much fats and hydrogenated soy oils as Americans do.

In spite of no scientific evidence of their efficacy, aggressive marketing of soy products as health foods that prevent heart disease and cancer, build strong bones, and help menopausal symptoms has led to annual sales increases in double digits. If you eat soy foods in any quantities produced by American food manufacturers, you should be aware you're being used as a laboratory test rat in a gigantic, uncontrolled dietary experiment that's never been tried before.

Asian people actually have the soy advantage when it comes to soy food consumption, but not because soy is in itself a health food. The Japanese people are among the highest consumers of soy in the world— mostly using traditional fermented or precipitated soy products—but they only consume around 8.6 grams daily. And Asian societies never ate soybeans at all, until they learned to cook and ferment the beans and enlist bacteria, fungi, and beneficial microorganisms to break down the proteins, fats, and starches into digestible amino acids, sugars, and fatty acids. The process of making miso, tempeh, aged soy sauces, and tofu results in a complete bio-chemical transformation that makes soy, in small amounts, into a healthy food.

The kind of soy eaten by Asian peoples also makes a difference, whether it is real soy or "soy protein," a manufactured product. When users of traditionally-made soy products eat tofu, they are only getting 8 to 15 grams of protein out of every 100 grams of product. The rest of the total is made up of fats and carbohydrates. But almost 90% of the soy products sold in America are fractionated soy proteins, such as *soy protein isolate,* yielding 80.7 grams of protein out of 100 grams, or *soy protein concentrate* with 58.1 grams out of 100 grams. In other words, if you eat a quarter of a pound of a garden burger or tofu sausage made from soy protein isolate, you're eating ten times as much soy as the average Japanese person does in a day.

At the same time the FDA has allowed a healthy heart claim to be displayed on soy products, the FDA also lists soy in its *Poisonous Plant Database.* You can access it yourself at: http://vm.cfsan.fea.gov/-djw/pltx.cgi?QUERY=SOY. If you search for "soy" in this FDA database, you'll find over 256 references to studies warning about endocrine disruption, carcinogenesis, growth problems, goiter, and amino acid and mineral deficiencies caused by soy products.

Soy-Based Baby Formula: A Very Bad Idea

One of the greatest dangers of eating soy foods that haven't been fermented in the traditional way is the use of soy-based formula for infants. If you're a parent, a grandparent, or even a friend—don't let anyone you know feed their baby soy formula. Currently, at least 25% of all baby formula sold in the U.S. is nutritionally deficient soy-based formula.

Once again the anti-cholesterol bandwagon has been rolled into play to dupe you into thinking soy baby formula is good for your child. There's an incredible difference between nutritionally inferior soy baby formula and mother's milk. Mother's breast milk is over 50% cholesterol, and cholesterol is essential for your child's development. Breast milk also contains a special enzyme that ensures babies can absorb all the cholesterol that's available. Why would nature design mother's milk this way, if it wasn't to give a baby large amounts of high quality cholesterol for optimum nourishment?

In traditional Chinese culture, pregnant women and nursing women used to eat as many as a dozen eggs daily to help their developing fetus obtain the best quality cholesterol to help with brain development. In the Andes Mountains, *quinoa*, the mother grain of the Incas, was also used in traditional Quechua culture to help nursing mothers produce large quantities of breast milk. Nutritionally, this also makes sense, as quinoa is extremely high in vitamins and minerals.

Why do developing babies need adequate amounts of high quality cholesterol and vitamins and minerals from natural sources? One good reason is that our brain is composed of over 60% cholesterol. Why would you want to short change a growing baby of a substance that's so critical for its development?

There are many other problems with soy formula that go much deeper than soy formula's lack of natural saturated fats and cholesterol. Because of the deep roots of soybean plants, they take up manganese, aluminum, cadmium and fluoride from the soil in amounts that vary according to the types of soybeans grown, the climate, and the processing of the beans. Aluminum levels as much as 100 times higher than those in breast milk can be found in soy baby formulas made from soy protein isolates, according to a study reported by the American Academy of Pediatrics. Aluminum interferes with metabolic processes and is linked to memory loss, dementia, and confusion, loss of coordination and digestive problems, including colic. Aluminum is most dangerous when combined with other toxic metals, such as manganese, fluoride, and natural plant estrogens—all of which are found in soy baby formula.

Fluoride and cadmium are also serious problems with soy baby formula. Cadmium is a toxic metal that has been linked to cancer, heart disease, diabetes, and reproductive problems. One study shows cadmium levels in soy formula are six times higher than dairy milk formula, and another shows levels are eight to fifteen times higher. Soy foods naturally contain fluoride from the soil, and the levels are sharply increased beyond allowable standards by using fluoridated water to make soy baby formula. Fluoride affects the central nervous system of infants and may exaggerate the effects of other neurotoxins, such as manganese, aluminum, cadmium and the plant estrogens in soybeans.

Manganese is a mineral which is essential in trace amounts in your diet. However, the problem with its accumulation in soybeans is that infants fed soy formula take in 75 to 80 times more manganese than breast fed infants. Breast milk contains 3 to 10 ug. Manganese per liter, cow's milk formula has 30 to 50 ug. and soy formula contains 200 to 300 ug. Young children and adults who ingest excess amounts of manganese can eliminate most of it, but infants don't have fully functioning livers and store the excess in their body and in their brains. The best test for mineral toxicities is hair analysis, and studies show that infants raised on soy formula have high levels of manganese in their scalp hair, which is a clear indicator of manganese toxicity.

In 2000, a conference was held in Irvine, California, at which leading toxicologists, pediatricians, and nutritionists warned that high manganese levels in soy baby formula could lead to behavioral problems, tendencies to violence, learning disabilities and attention deficit disorders. As far back as 1983, Phillip J. Collipp, M.D., a pediatrician at Nassau County Medical Center, correlated high manganese levels in children with learning disabilities and observed that the use of soy-based infant formula might be the single most important factor in a child developing ADD (Attention Deficit Disorder) or ADHD (Attention Deficit Hyperactivity Disorder). Hair samples from youths convicted of felonies also consistently show elevated levels of manganese.

As soy formula manufacturers are largely in denial regarding the manganese problem, a few citizens and scientists are beginning to ring alarm bells. Recently, Everett L. "Red" Hodges, the founder of the Violence Research Institute helped set up informational hearings before the California Public Safety Committee. Scientists who have done animal research testified on the mounting body of evidence that the high manganese content of soy formula is a factor in violent crime and behavioral disorders in young people. One of the only manufacturers of soy products who have done anything about the manganese problem is Lumen Foods, which recently posted the following warning on its cartons of soy milk: *WARNING: Soymilk may be detrimental to infants under six months of age. It contains manganese at levels important to human nutrition but over 50 times the level found in mother's breast milk.*

There have been some sad stories of infants admitted to hospitals whose parents were vegans or vegetarians and who tried to substitute soy milks for soy formulas. Both Edensoy and Soy-Moo soy milks have been implicated in hospital admissions of mal-nourished children. Stuart Nightingale, M.D., and Assistant Commissioner for Health Affairs at the FDA issued a warning about the use of soy milks as baby formula in 1990, stating they were "grossly lacking in the nutrients needed for infants." Dr. Nightingale also asked all soy milk manufacturers to put warning labels on soymilks so they would not be used as formula substitutes. Obviously, almost no soy milk manufacturers put warnings on their labels. Mostly what I see on the carton of Silk brand vanilla soymilk on my desktop (I'm using it as a paperweight) is the health claims that it's high in calcium, low in fat, and "may help reduce the risk of osteoporosis and may help prevent heart disease."

Soy Foods and Your Hormones

Another health menace in consuming improperly processed American soy foods is their large load of phytoestrogens. Structurally, these plant hormones are similar enough to human hormones that they bind with estrogen receptor sites on cells throughout your body. The fact that these "natural" soy phytoestrogens can actually replace your body's hormones has led researchers to propose that they can be used for cancer prevention, lowering cholesterol levels, and as estrogen substitutes in hormone replacement therapies.

The natural phytoestrogens in soybeans are called *isoflavones* and they exist in over 70 plants, but their highest concentration is found in soybeans. Research isn't conclusive, but there appear to be strong correlations between the use of soy formula and the rising incidence of thyroid diseases and thyroid cancer, especially among young people. Both soy foods and soybean formulas contain high concentrations of soy isoflavones that act as *goitrogens,* which are substances blocking the synthesis of thyroid hormones. Only extraction by chemical solvents can de-activate these isoflavones, and the soy industry has resisted doing this—even for soy products manufactured for infant formulas. Vegans who use soy as their principal food, infants on soy formula, and men or women who are self-medicating with soy isoflavones supplements have been identified as being a high risk population for soy-induced thyroid disease by the United Kingdom's Committee on Toxicity.

Many studies on laboratory animals and increasing numbers of reports from parents and pediatricians also suggest that the plant estrogens in soy baby formula can seriously damage later sexual development and reproductive health of infants fed with soy formula. One of America's most progressive advocates for good health, the Weston A. Price Foundation in Washington D.C., is currently lobbying for a ban on the sale of all soy infant formulas except by a doctor's prescription. The Swiss Federal Health Service has estimated that parents who feed their babies soy formula are giving them the hormonal equivalent of 3 to 5 birth control pills each day.

The same sort of risks to infants from consuming soy formula extend into the womb and affect the development of fetuses. It has been well documented that adult males who consume foods rich in soy estrogens (American style soy foods) have reported lower testosterone and higher estrogen levels. So it shouldn't be a surprise that estrogen-like soy isoflavones can suppress or interfere with an unborn baby boy's testosterone production. (The development of female genitals in the womb is largely independent of hormones, but proper male development will only occur if male hormones are present. That's why there are eight times more birth defects involving sex organs among males than females.)

Currently, there are increasing numbers of baby boys being born with genital abnormalities, such as *hypospadias*. This is a disorder in which the meatus (the urethra's opening) appears somewhere on the underside of the penis and is located anywhere between the tip of the penis and the scrotum. Usually, it occurs about an inch back from the tip and can be repaired surgically, so it doesn't interfere with sex or urination. The numbers of hypospadia cases are increasing in the European Union and in the U.S. and now occur in one of out 125 live births. A recent study showed vegetarian mothers were five times more likely to give birth to a baby boy with hypospadias than a mother who was an omnivore.

Many of the problems of male fetuses who are estrogenized in the womb might not manifest until puberty or adulthood. When male hormones necessary to program the reproductive system are absent (the right molecule at the right time), demasculinizing effects can occur throughout the body. Environmental estrogens (plastics) and plant phytoestrogens (soy isoflavones) have been demonstrated to alter development of key brain cells controlling sexual behavior, reproduction, and possibly even sexual preference.

Soy formula is extremely bad news for baby girls, too. In baby girls who develop normally, estrogen levels will double in the first month of life, then decline and stay at low levels until puberty. The effects of plastics in the environment that create estrogen mimicking effects in the body and plant phytoestrogens (from soy products) appear to be an important factor in the alarming numbers of girls entering puberty at an early age. One per cent of all girls now have signs of puberty, such as pubic hair or breast development, before age three. By age eight, almost 15% of Caucasian girls and slightly over 48% of African-American girls have one or both of these characteristics of puberty.

It's a fact that black people experience puberty slightly earlier than whites, but these wildly disproportionate statistics are a recent phenomenon. It's generally accepted that early puberty is caused by exposure to the increasing numbers of estrogens and estrogen mimickers, such as plastics, pesticides, commercial animal products (DES) and soy phytoestrogens. It's well known that African-American woman are the primary beneficiaries of the WIC (Women, Infants, and Children) Federal government program established in 1974 that provides free infant formula to teen-age and low income mothers. Because of the possibility of lactose-intolerance and of government contracts with food manufacturers and suppliers, African-American babies have a high probability of receiving soy baby formula from WIC programs.

I've spent a lot of time informing you of the dangers of soy to fetuses and babies because I was horrified to discover such a defective product that's so widely used with so little knowledge of the detrimental effects to the young. A lot of the alarming information has come from health departments in foreign countries such as the U.K., or Switzerland. Why can't our own Food and Drug Administration take measures to protect the very young in our country?

Soy Milk No Substitute

I'm fortunate that I didn't consume much soy milk in my short career as a soy milk drinker. Soy milk sales continue to rocket off the charts—their sales have been a food marketers dream—White Wave, Silk, etc., have been some of the best marketed products in American history. In 2005, soy milk sales climbed past $1 billion. A lot of American soy milk drinkers would be surprised to know there is no history of this beverage being consumed in Asian societies. Soy milk was only a step in the process of making tofu. The earliest reference to soy milk in Asian Culture only dates to 1866.

There's nothing natural about soy milk. It's a machine made product in which the beans are soaked, ground, cooked, and strained to make soy milk. New methods speed up the traditional process, but the high pH of the soaking solution and pressure cooking destroys large amounts of the vitamins and amino acids.

Soy milk needs more than processing to make it palatable. The aftertaste and beany flavor comes from oxidized phospholipids (rancid lecithin), oxidized fatty acids (rancid soy oil), anti-nutrients such as saponins, and soy estrogens (soy isoflavones). The soy estrogens are so bitter tasting, they make your mouth dry and the only way the soy industry can make the milk drinkable is to remove or chemically neutralize the very toxins (soy isoflavones) they are promoting as being beneficial in lowering cholesterol and preventing cancer.

The best ways the soy industry has found to make soy milk drinkable is to add strong flavors, such as vanilla, chocolate and/or sugar. Who would think your soy milk is high in sugar? Most of them are—they range from 4 to 16 grams of sugar per 8 oz. serving.

All soymilks are fortified with calcium, vitamin D, and other vitamins and minerals lacking in soybeans. These supplements are cheap, mass produced products and the vitamin D^2 added to soymilk is a supplement the dairy industry quietly quit adding to milk many years ago. (Vitamin D^2 has been linked to allergic reactions, coronary heart disease, and hyperactivity.) Low fat or "lite" soymilks are made from soy protein islolate, instead of full-fat soybeans. Because soymilk made with soy protein isolate needs to have some oil added, canola oil is added, because the soy industry knows the public doesn't perceive soy oil as healthy.

Soybean Oil Damages Health

I've saved the greatest possible danger to your health from soybeans to the end of this mass production soybean story. It's, of course, the danger to your health from eating the oxidized cholesterol found in rancid soybean oils, hydrogenated soy oil, and trans-fats. Contrary to what millions of people believe, your body needs high quality fats and cholesterol for energy, mineral absorption, hormone production, and to build flexible, high functioning cell membranes. The most damaging oils to your health are not healthy tropical oils, like coconut oil or saturated fats from animals, but refined and processed polyunsaturated oils that come from plants. Some of the worst of them come from soybeans.

Soybean oil is at its healthiest when it's left intact as whole beans in fermented soy products, such as miso and tempeh. The soy fats in soymilk and tofu are also safe, although the load of phytoestrogens, phytates, goitrogens, hormones and anti-nutrients make these products unsuitable to eat in any substantial quantities.

Close to 80% of the vegetable oils consumed in the US are made from soybeans. This includes bottled vegetable oils, margarine, shortening (Crisco), salad dressings, and oil for frying. Nearly all of this oil is fully or partially hydrogenated.

Almost all the experts are in agreement that hydrogenated oils and the trans fats created by hydrogenation are bad for you. The industry has a real problem because labeling of trans fats is now a law, and trans fats are in almost everything on the shelf in the American supermarket. "Soybean oil, if hydrogenated, is not recommended for daily use," says Neil Solomon, M.D., in his book *Soy Smart Health*. In other words— almost all the food products in your average supermarket shouldn't be eaten on a daily basis!

The problem with soy bean oils is they contain *lipoxydase* which catalyzes oxidation and forms free radicals. Free radicals make oils go rancid—they also make our bodies go rancid too. Eating rancid oils starts chain reactions causing cell destruction, damage to our DNA, accelerated aging, and disease.

Help is on the way for soybean growers—new versions of soybeans are being tested that are low in *linolenic acid* (the source of lipoxydase) that won't need hydrogenation. Are they safe or good for you? Time will tell....given the many problems that have resulted from our technological quick fixes to problems—it might be wise to do some extensive testing before they're widely used in food manufacturing.

Soy Sauce and Miso, American Style

I still enjoy eating small amounts of aged miso and tofu, and I've learned to appreciate soy sauces made in the traditional way. Before World War II in Japan, soy sauce (*shoyu*) was made from soybeans that had undergone a long fermenting process. The soybeans were roasted and blended with cracked wheat, then spores from an Aspergillus mold were added. The culture was grown for three days and mixed with salt water, then brewed in fermentation tanks for six to eighteen months. This process has over 600 years of development in the tradition of making a distinctive, high quality natural product. Other traditional types of soy sauce are *shiro* and *tamari*.

Contrast this with how most soy sauces you've eaten all your life in America are manufactured: Soybean meal and/or corn starches are cooked with acid based chemicals for 8 to 12 hours and then the brew is neutralized with sodium carbonate. The resulting dark liquid is a chemical soy sauce. Sometimes it's mixed with some traditional fermented soy sauce to make it into a semi-chemical soy sauce. Preservatives, pasteurization, artificial colors, sweeteners, and flavor enhancers, such as MSG, are then added—then it's off to the table at your local Chinese restaurant! These formulations often contain dangerous chemicals such as *furanones, ethyl carbonate*, and *chloropropanols*.

Miso production is a similar story to soy sauce production. High quality misos are aged for one to three years, and are only made from natural whole ingredients. Made in the traditional way, they are never pasteurized, because the process destroys enzymes that aid digestion. Quick misos were first produced about 1960. They are made in only 3 to 21 days, are pasteurized, and have sweeteners, bleaches, food colorings, MSG and sorbic acid added to them. These industrial grade misos were implicated with sharply increased prostate cancer risk in a study from 1979 of 122,261 Japanese men.

As I said early on in my story of soy, about traditional soy products vs. the New American style soy products—for your good health, you should only eat soy foods in small amounts and eat them as much as possible prepared in the traditional Asian manner. They are not a health food, nor are they a suitable substitute for healthier foods that might contain cholesterol and saturated fat. The dangers of soy outweigh those of foods mistakenly believed to be the heavy hitters in causing heart disease.

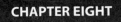
How To Avoid Cancer

In our culture, we readily accept the fact that cancer kills millions of people each year. What most of us don't know is that cancer was very rare as recently as 100 years ago. Cancer has always been a disease that can kill you when you in your twilight years, but only recently has cancer become a disease that can kill you in the prime of life.

There are a lot of doctors out there who shrug their shoulders and try to tell you that genetics will determine whether or not you get cancer. This attitude directly contradicts the authors of a major review on cancer and diet, done in 1981 for the U.S. Congress, that estimated genetics determines only about 2 to 3% of total cancer risk. And of course, toxins in the environment are a factor in cancer, but according to the research, they only account for a small amount of cancers.

Few people realize that cancer, like heart disease, is primarily a disease caused by a poor diet lacking in the right types and amounts of nutrients. Most cancer incidence is also strongly correlated with having a weak immune and lymph system, both of which don't function well enough to protect you.

Surprisingly enough, both cancer and heart disease were completely unknown in primitive populations that had the good fortune of not eating the modern processed foods Americans eat. In this chapter, I'm going to show you how deficient our health is compared to our primitive' ancestors who ate a diet rich in phyto-chemicals, vitamins and minerals. I'm also going to give a basic dietary regimen for men that will greatly decrease the odds of getting prostate cancer. Prostate cancer also has strong correlations with vitamin and mineral deficiencies. But first, some words of advice about breast cancer and the food women eat in America.

Breast Cancer and Hormones in Food

It's a shocking statistic that the rate of breast cancer has increased over 50% since 1965. I read a lot of dietary and health advice for women on how to avoid breast cancer, but only one thing I discovered had enough scientific integrity behind it for me to recommend it. *Avoid consuming meat produced in the USA that isn't certified organic.*

All Americans, from birth to death, consume unknown amounts of synthetic hormones and antibiotics given to livestock in their feed, and there is absolutely no warning or labeling to protect you. This little publicized health issue is caused by feeding beef cattle abnormal amounts of corn, soybeans, and grain. This practice causes severe gastro-intestinal problems for the animals, and they often have liver problems. Also, when cattle stand and lay in their own manure in crowded feed-lots day and night, they're susceptible to infections. Pumping them full of antibiotics, steroids, and hormones is American agri-business's shake-and-bake solution to this ongoing problem.

The European Union doesn't allow American beef imports for very good reasons. The question that should be asked isn't, *Why won't the Europeans buy our hormone and antibiotic laden beef?* But rather: *Why should we allow hormone laden beef, poultry, pork and milk to be sold to Americans and Canadians?*

We now know that synthetic hormones in the food supply are strongly linked to breast cancer. Their usage in animal feed is of serious concern, as the recent statistical linkage between breast cancer and synthetic hormone replacement is now well documented. Hormones are one of many potential health hazards involved in the production of industrial beef, pork, chicken and factory milk. Some of the others are the thousands of other food additives, antibiotics, pesticides and drugs that have entered the food supply due to lax regulations and lack of enforcement by the USDA and the FDA.

The synthetic hormones given to livestock are probably the most likely reason for the soaring levels of all reproductive cancers in the U.S. Since 1950, breast cancer is up 55%, prostate cancer is up 190%, and testicular cancer is up 120%. This is one facet of your health that needs more research in order for me to speak with authority. We don't know what percentage of these breast cancers are caused by synthetic hormones in the food chain from livestock consumption, and what percentage are caused by natural plant estrogens from soy products or estrogen mimicking plastics in the environment. For your good health, all synthetic estrogens are to be avoided.

Of course, you should also avoid getting dioxin carcinogens from plastics, which are known to cause breast cancer, by using products like Saran Wrap in microwave ovens. You should never put plastic products in microwave ovens or freeze plastic water bottles in your freezer, as both of these practices release dioxin into your food or drinking water, according to a publication from John Hopkins Medical Center, *Cancer News,* in December of 2004.

One of the biggest disappointments of my research for this book was that I was unable to find a dietary regimen for women to avoid breast cancer or develop a program for hormone replacement after menopause. I'm not sure our government is up to the task, either. Given the current state of affairs in Washington, D.C., I'm not sure federal funding would accomplish anything. The best hope for women is for private foundations to research breast cancer and develop a safe, healthy program for hormone replacement.

Cancer in the Ancient World

Cancer is so common now, it's hard to believe it was largely unknown among primitive peoples. Even though it was extremely rare, cancer is an ancient disease and it was the Greek philosopher Hippocrates, the father of medicine, who gave cancer its name. Even before Hippocrates, evidence of cancerous tumors has been found by modern researchers in dinosaur bones and Egyptian mummies.

Surprisingly enough, Hippocrates was also the first to make the diet-cancer connection. He believed that cancer was caused by a poor diet and lack of exercise. Ironically enough, his hunch was probably right in many ways. A good diet and being active is one of the best things you can do to lessen your risk of cancer. A lot of the practices of modern medicine and Big Pharma would come to a screeching halt if they obeyed what Hippocrates said thousands of years ago: *First, Do No Harm.*

In our modern world, where so many of us aren't physically active, we've lost touch with the natural world and the power and strength that comes from being connected with nature. The feats of physical strength performed on a daily basis by our primitive ancestors, show what sort of a body you can have if you eat natural foods and exercise vigorously. None of us are going to perform acts of physical prowess like the ones I'm about to describe—but do the best you can—and be active as much as possible.

Before their genocide in the 19th century by British colonists, Tasmanian aborigines were observed throwing 15 foot long spears a distance of 250 feet. They regularly hit animals at distances of 180 feet. On the Pacific Coast of western North America, the Nootka Indians who hunted California gray whales into the late 1890s, routinely harpooned these giant whales from small, hide covered, eight-man boats. As few as two boats, powered by cedar wood oars and muscle power, would tow a whale back to shore, sometimes rowing over ten miles.

Unlike muscle strength, which has declined greatly since the agricultural revolution, our potential for aerobic fitness has undoubtedly changed little since the Industrial Revolution, which is less than 200 years old. We have the genetic potential to engage in the same sort of aerobic fitness such as that displayed by Native American runners in pre-Columbian times.

Within 24 hours of Hernando Cortez's landing at Chianiztlan on the Mexican coast in 1519, native runners had described Cortez's strange ships, bearded men, guns and horses to the Aztec ruler, Montezuma, 260 miles away. These same runners routinely supplied Montezuma's dinner tables with fresh red snapper from the Gulf of Mexico. In North America, Iroquois runners would travel the 240 mile distance along the Iroquois (Haudenosanee) Trail in four days. In exceptional circumstances, they would do it in three days and cover as much as 90 miles in a day!

In America, where affluence and obesity has settled in upon tens of millions of us, we no longer know that our birthright as human beings is to be strong, healthy, and disease free. Few have any understanding what a culture of weak and sick people we've become. Cancer and heart disease have been accepted by millions as simply being some of the travails of life that befall you as you age. Genetically, you are little different than Native Americans who were physically fit and strong and to whom the diseases of civilization were extremely rare. It is your diet that makes you ill, and few realize how deadly and toxic the modern diet of processed foods is.

Cancer: A Disease of Civilization

The first awareness that cancer is a disease of civilization began with the publication of a monograph in 1843 by the French medical researcher Stanislaus Tanchou. Tanchou proved statistically that cancer deaths were increasing in Paris, and he came to the realization that cancer is "a disease of civilization." because cancer rates were so much higher in urban areas than rural areas. He formulated his observations into Tanchou's Doctrine, which states cancer increases in direct proportion to the civilization of a nation.

The first reliable statistics on cancer from Wales and Scotland in the 1830s showed the cancer rate to be 166 per million per year. By 1905, these figures had increased over five times. In the mid 1900s, cancer rates began to rise sharply with increased prosperity and increased consumption of white flour, sugar, hydrogenated oils, and processed foods.

Around the turn of the century, educated medical personnel began to live and work among vanishing tribes of indigenous peoples around the world. Everywhere they brought back the news that disease such as heart disease and cancer were almost unknown among primitive peoples.

John Le Conte, MD (1818-1891), who was the first president of the University of California, embraced Tanchou's Doctrine, and his interest led ship's surgeons, anthropologists, and missionaries to search for cancer among the native peoples of Alaska, Canada, and Labrador. For almost 75 years, not a single case of cancer was discovered by experienced, competent medical examiners.

The Hunza, who lived in remote valleys of the Himalayas in Kashmir, were also much studied starting in 1910 by many observers including Robert McCarrison, Major General of the Indian Health Service. His seven years of study led him to conclude cancer was almost non-existent in this population.

Similar stories came back from early travelers in Asia and Africa who lived with native peoples eating a traditional diet. Albert Schweitzer MD, the famous Nobel laureate, wrote in his autobiography, *Out of My Life and Thought*:

> *On my arrival in Gabon in 1913, I was astonished to encounter no case of cancer... The absence of cancer seemed to me due to the difference in nutrition of the natives as compared with the Europeans....In the course of the years, we have seen cases of cancer in growing numbers in our region. My observations incline me to attribute this to the fact that the natives were living more and more after the manner of the whites...I have naturally been interested in any research tracing the occurrence of cancer to some defect in our mode of nutrition.*

Dr. Joseph Romig, an experienced surgeon who traveled widely among the Inuit and the Indians in northern Canada early in the last century, reported that in his 36 years of contact with these people, he never saw a case of malignant disease, although cancer frequently occurred when they became modernized. Romig recorded the native diets he observed among the Inuit in the book *Dogteam Doctor: The Story of Dr. Romig* by Eva Greenslit Anderson published in 1943:

> *The food was in a wooden dish...mostly game and fish. Dried smoked salmon was much used and other dried fish. Seal and fish oil was much in demand. Their food was cooked mostly by boiling, and was rather rare. They ate as well, especially in winter, raw frozen fish and raw meat. They kept some wild cranberries for the favored dish of akutok, made of lean meat and of seal or fish oil, mixed with warm tallow, sprinkled with cranberries, stirred and hardened with a little snow. ... On this diet the people were strong, and did not get scurvy...they did not have gastric ulcer, cancer, diabetes, malaria, or typhoid fever, or the common diseases of childhood known so well among whites. For the most part, they were a happy, carefree people.*

Inuit diet and lifestyle changed dramatically when gold was discovered nearby, and with the coming of missions and government schools. Dr. Romig wrote, "These people have changed from the old way, to eating pancakes with syrup and canned goods from the store." He added that with the change in their diet, both young and old alike had dental problems, and they became vulnerable to the diseases of white people.

Perhaps the most unusual and interesting book in the health and nutrition field was *Nutrition and Physical Degeneration* by Weston A. Price, published in 1939. In his writing, the Cleveland dentist describes his investigation of the health of primitive peoples in the 1930s. He and his wife Florence traveled worldwide, extensively examining the dental hygiene and dietary habits of isolated Irish fisher folk, Pacific Islanders, Australian Aborigines, Africans, and North and South American tribal peoples. Dr. Price's research showed that primitive peoples everywhere enjoyed good health until they turned to the civilized diet of processed foods, sugar and white flour. When they adapted the food habits of the modern world, their dental hygiene and overall health began to worsen with each generation.

Dr. Price was the first to put his attention into figuring out why savages had such excellent teeth, instead of studying why our culture has such poor teeth. Dr. Price was a strong advocate of the healing powers of cod liver oil, butter, raw milk, raw foods, organ meats, fish eggs, coconut oils, fresh fish, poultry and meat. What he found was that foods used by isolated primitive peoples contained *four times* the water soluble vitamins, minerals and calcium and over *ten times* the fat soluble vitamins. His work is carried on by some of the most progressive nutritionists in America at the Weston A. Price Foundation. You can get in touch with them on the internet at www.westonaprice. org. Another good source of reputable medical advice online is Dr. Joe Mercola, whom you can reach at www.mercola.com.

Recently, epidemiologists including Graham Colditz and Leslie Frazier of the Harvard School of Public Health have reached the conclusion that the vast majority of cancers—at least 65% and possibly as much as 80%—can be prevented using fairly simple methods. Obviously, eliminating this deadly disease from our lives or at least delaying it for many years would give us a lot less sorrow and more joy in our lives.

Failure of Cancer Treatment

The focus of this chapter is almost entirely upon preventing cancer, as cancer treatments don't work nearly as well as the medical establishment would lead you to believe. The primary medical treatments for cancer are the treatments developed by research during World War II: radiation and chemotherapy, still the cornerstones of almost all cancer treatments. Essentially, our modern treatments consist of cutting, (surgery), burning (radiation), and poisoning (chemotherapy).

Chemotherapy "works" by poisoning the cancer cells in your body. Big Pharma sells chemo treatments with the full knowledge that all other cells in your body will be damaged, too. Instead of strengthening your body's immune system to help it fight the cancer cells, chemotherapy will paralyze and weaken your immune system. The side effects of chemotherapy require you to use many other medications, such as cortisone, painkillers, antibiotics, plasma replacement drugs, and many more. The last few weeks or months of treatment is a veritable gold mine for Big Pharma. It's one of the reasons why 10% of patients account for 69% of medical costs each year, according to an article in the *Wall Street Journal,* January 31, 2006.

You're not alone in being a victim of poorly thought out, debilitating treatments like chemotherapy—the same fate can befall you even if you're a President or a King. In 1999, King Hussein of Jordan had some of the best possible treatment for his leukemia (blood cancer) at the famed Mayo Clinic in Rochester, Minnesota. The chemotherapy destroyed his bone marrow, which often happens, and a bone marrow transplant was ordered. King Hussein didn't survive the bone marrow transplant. His case is just one more where chemotherapy killed him quicker than the disease would have. If kings can be so seriously misinformed and maltreated, what odds do you have of getting good medical treatment?

In the 1960s, there were some voices of dissent against medical orthodoxy, such as Francisco Contreras, M.D., who wrote *Health in the 21ˢᵗ Century, Will Doctors Survive?* He wrote of many doctors who discovered that patients not subjected to conventional therapies often had longer life expectancies than those undergoing medical treatments for cancer. His observations was validated 20 years later in *Scientific American,* when in November of 1985, an article stated "chemotherapy treatments for cancer, which are given to about 50% of cancer patients, helped no more than 5% of them." We no longer have many rebellious, independent-minded young doctors like those in the 1960s. I'm afraid those who question the system have been replaced by young, financially well-off doctors only too eager to get into their BMWs and head for the golf course.

My family ran into the chemotherapy question in 2004 at Cottage Hospital in Santa Barbara, when my then 78 year old mother, Mary, underwent breast cancer surgery. Her illness was an iatrogenic illness (physician caused), because her breast cancer developed as a result of using Premarin, an estrogen replacement drug, for over 20 years. After a successful surgery, family members had a conference with her physician to discuss her follow-up treatment.

What the doctor said was a real eye-opener. He recommended chemotherapy, but when we questioned him about this, he revealed statistics showed for a 78 year old woman, only 1% of patients in her age group would derive *any benefit* whatsoever from chemotherapy.

My mother didn't have chemotherapy. She had an excellent outcome, and three years later she's doing better than ever. However, the oncologist at Cottage Hospital wasn't happy with her decision and pestered her to have chemotherapy *treatment.* Thanks, but no thanks! Who, at age 78, would undergo such a debilitating treatment, with such low odds of receiving any benefit from it? Obviously, many would, if they didn't have family members there to ask questions and use some common sense in seeking medical treatment. Needless to say, second and third opinions are often an excellent idea in the modern medical world.

American Cancer Society: Worse than Useless

It's probably a good time to mention a few things I discovered about The American Cancer Society while researching this book. First of all, I'd like to thank the many well intentioned people who've taken part in events such as *Run for the Cure,* fund raising efforts, and the annual sales of daffodils. I admire your great American spirit of doing something collectively to try and help out with the terrible problem of cancer.

However, the American Cancer Society is a worse than useless vehicle to do anything to help Americans with the cancer situation in our country. Many, many billions of dollars have been spent with *zero* results since the War on Cancer was declared in 1971. The American Cancer Society has accomplished *next to nothing* in this so called War on Cancer. The way the world's wealthiest non-profit is operated, it's a no-brainer that it's doomed to failure—just like the Vietnam War, the War on Drugs, and the failed War in Iraq.

Despite the tremendous amounts of evidence that cancer can be prevented by diet, the American Cancer Society continues to spend money only on diagnosis and treatment research, mostly designed to benefit big pharmaceutical companies. The non-profit status of ACS is in sharp contrast with its large financial reserves, extremely high overhead and expenses, and large contributions to political parties. Helping out someone you know with cancer would do a great deal more than giving money to the American Cancer Society.

Americans are a generous people and every year they give large sums of money to the American Cancer Society that *accomplish nothing* and actually hinder and repress many promising alternative cancer therapies. In 1992, *The Chronicle of Philanthropy* reported the American Cancer Society was "more interested in accumulating wealth than in saving lives." At that time, urgent fund raising appeals stated the ACS needed more funds to support cancer programs, when they actually had more than $750 million in cash and real estate on hand.

The same researchers discovered that in Arizona, less than 10% of funds were spent on community cancer support services; in California the figure was 11%, and it was less than 9% in Missouri. They figured for every dollar that was spent on community services, approximately $6.40 was spent on salaried compensation and overhead. In all ten states investigated, salaries and fringe benefits for staff were the largest component of their budgets, which was surprising in light of their many appeals stating the urgent and critical need for donations to provide direct services to assist cancer patients. Nationally, less than 16% of all funds raised are actually spent on direct services to cancer patients.

What the American Cancer Society doesn't want you to know about is its many complicated relationships with Big Pharma, the chemical industries, and the medical/industrial complex. Large amounts of funds from the American Cancer Society are spent each year on sponsored research trials of patented, profitable cancer drugs. As if Big Pharma needs help from the American Cancer Society? It's a noble and generous American desire to help out with America's cancer problem—but my suggestion is to find a better forum than volunteering or donating money to organizations as useless as the American Cancer Society.

The words of two-time Nobel Prize winner, Dr. Linus Pauling are an apt summation of the progress being made by the War on Cancer. In 1989, he said, "Everyone should know that most cancer research is largely a fraud and that the major cancer research organizations are derelict in their duties to the people who support them."

Your Lymph System: Front Line of Defense

One of the most important things anyone can do to reduce your risk of cancer is to make sure your lymph system is in good condition. Western medicine pays little or no attention to your lymph system, yet caring for it has always been important in Asian medicine. In the next chapter, I'm going to go into great detail how nutritional fasting cleans out and gives a strong boost to your lymph system and your liver.

Your lymph system is so important for your good health that you have three times as much lymph fluid as blood. Shouldn't that tell you something of the importance of your lymph system? Millions upon millions of tiny nodes in your lymph system work overtime guarding your body against intrusion from dangerous substances. Placed end to end, all the lymph vessels in your body would stretch out over 100,000 miles. Unlike your blood system, your lymph system carries waste material away from your cells, making it your frontline of defense in protecting you from toxins. More than 99% of soluble toxins (antigens) are trapped in your lymph nodes.

Many of us who grew up in the 1950s had our tonsils removed and consequently have medically comprised lymph systems. It's now well known by medicine that your tonsils are an important ring of lymph tissue providing powerful protection at the openings between your oral and nasal cavities against bacteria and other harmful materials. Unlike in the '50s and '60s, your tonsils are no longer regarded as a vestigial organ. Perhaps the tonsillitis many of us had that led to having our tonsils removed was a natural reaction to the food additives, chemicals, sugars, and hydrogenated oils introduced to the national diet in the 1950s.

Also you should know that Hodgkin's disease is three times more prevalent among those who've had their tonsils removed. This is another shocking statistic, like the fact that men who've had vasectomies are three times more likely to get prostate cancer, as reported in *Medical Journal*, August of 1989. I have tried to point out a few of these failures of our command-and-control system of medicine along the way, encouraging you to be careful taking advice from medical experts.

The best way to help out your lymph system is by taking adequate amounts of anti-oxidants, such as vitamin C, natural B vitamins, such as those in brewer's yeast, and avoiding hydrogenated oils. Cellulite tissue is a symptom of a bad diet that causes lymph fluid to be trapped in the cells. It's a sign you need to make big changes in your diet. Drinking lots of fluids and being physically active is critical to the functioning of your lymph system.

Prostrate Cancer and Diet

You need a high functioning lymph system and liver to help you avoid one of the most common cancers for men—prostate cancer. If you're a man, you need to be pro-active and use preventative nutrients to avoid prostate cancer. The levels of prostate cancer in America are probably at some of the highest levels recorded in any society, and much of it can be avoided by dietary means.

Once again, on the medical side we're in the process of finding many of the tests for prostate cancer are notoriously unreliable and are far less useful than they've been represented. The PSA test, the most common test, is now known to have a high false positive rate, and about 70% of the time it incorrectly suggests a man has cancer, according to the National Cancer Institute. Most men who undergo a biopsy (with subsequent risk of infection and scar tissue) often don't get decisive results either.

There is no guarantee that surgery will find cancer, either. Sloan-Kettering Hospital recently did a study where they looked at 2,000 patients whose prostates were removed in the last four years after biopsies said they had cancer. In more than 30% of cases, the prostate either had microscopic amounts of cancer that weren't life threatening—or none at all! Apparently, cells removed in biopsies had cancer, but the rest of the prostate was cancer free. It is known from a recent study at Wayne State University in Detroit that 8% of 1,027 men in their twenties who died of other causes had small amounts of prostate cancer. The percentage rose with each decade, and over 80% of men in their seventies had microscopic cancers in their prostates discovered during autopsies.

These diagnostic and decision-making problems are coming up because new medical imaging and detection methods are finding cancer where they were unable to before. What they're starting to find is that it's not that unusual for many people in our culture to have cancer in their bodies—it appears *most* people have some cancer cells in their body. This is a startling *new* idea being proposed by a growing number of medical researchers.

Now that I've told you all the confusing problems of falling into the camp of being a prostate patient, hopefully I've sharpened your interest in using nutritional tools to avoid getting prostate cancer.

We have excellent nutritional substances to help keep your prostate healthy. The first step is making sure you take adequate amounts of the mineral *selenium*. Take 100 to 200 mg. daily. There—you've just reduced the odds of having an enlarged prostate or getting prostate cancer by 63%. Do you feel better, knowing that? You have also drastically reduced your chances of many other types of cancers by making sure you take adequate levels of selenium.

Next, make sure you take a daily vitamin that has adequate levels of the mineral *zinc*. The reason for this is your prostate contains more zinc than any other gland in your body. We also know that a diseased prostate has very low concentrations of zinc, and that vitamin C works much better when adequate zinc is present. It's an interesting fact that oysters contain the highest amounts of zinc of any natural foods. Oysters have four times as much zinc as wheat germ—which is in number two position. Oysters have always had the reputation of being an aphrodisiac and a rejuvenator, and there's good medical reasons for their folk reputation. Oysters, mussels, and clams are all excellent foods for prostate health.

Probably the single most important nutritional supplement you can take also has its roots in folk medicine. Folklore from Bulgaria, Germany, Turkey and the Ukraine says eating a handful of pumpkin seeds every day gives men increased virility and helps with prostate functions. When the medical University in Vienna investigated these claims, they found that prostatic hypertrophy (enlarged prostate) was almost non-existent in areas where men ate a handful of pumpkin seeds every day. Pumpkin seeds were also used in primitive cultures by Native Americans and Africans for prostate health. These seeds are extremely high in essential fatty acids and it turns out your prostate tissue is high in fatty acids too. A teaspoon of pumpkin seed oil daily is also beneficial for prostate function. So eat a handful of pumpkin seeds every day for good prostate health—preferably raw. Pumpkin seeds also turn out to be high in zinc.

Another traditional herbal remedy for prostrate health is to take pills containing saw palmetto berry extract. Make sure you take at least 160 mg. daily of standardized extract containing at least 85 to 95% (135-152 mg.) fatty acids with active sterols. This works well for most men. Recently, there have been some studies stating saw palmetto berry extracts have no effect on prostate problems in men with moderate to severe prostate enlargement. My personal take on this is it's hard to argue with the 2.5 million men who take this drug and believe it has substantial effects.

Were these recent studies medical dis-information underwritten by business interests eager to sell you Big Pharma-style prostate medicine like Proscar? I don't know—it would be a good subject for the FDA to investigate. In the current political climate, I'm not going to hold my breath and wait for the FDA to investigate anything.

Other foods which are good for your prostate are the oils found in mackerel, sardines, flaxseed and grape seed oils. Also, *lycopenes* found in tomatoes and *sulforaphanes* found in broccoli, cabbage, and *cauliflowers* are good for prostate function. The mineral boron, green tea, exposure to sunlight, and vitamin E are also excellent for prostate health.

Some Final Words About Cancer Causes

When you realize how well these natural nutrients work in

preventing a disease like prostate cancer, you realize how apt the words of Dr. Paavo Airola are from his book, written over 30 years ago, entitled, *How to Get Well*: "Cancer is a disease of civilization. It is the end result of health-destroying living and eating habits, which result in biochemical imbalance, and physical and chemical irritation of the tissues."

Dr. Airola also makes the assertion that excess acidity in your system is the basis of many cancers, and while I don't have good science to back it up, it certainly rings true with me. "In the healing of disease, when the patient usually has acidosis (over-acidity), the higher the ratio of alkaline elements in the diet, the faster will be the recovery," he wrote.

Over acidity is caused by eating a diet high in acid foods. The most acidic substances in your diet, ranging from the most acidic to the least are: Tobacco, drugs, medications, alcohol, salt, coffee, fried meats, spices, white meats, sugar, dairy products, eggs and whole grains. Maintaining a more alkaline environment in your body requires eating from the most alkaline foods, such as figs, lima beans, apricots, spinach, beet greens, raisins, almonds, carrots, dates, celery, cucumber, cantaloupe, lettuce, potatoes, cabbage, grapefruit, tomatoes, peaches, apples, grapes, bananas, watermelon, millet, brazil nuts, coconuts and buckwheat. "All vegetable and fruit juices are high alkaline," states Dr. Airola. "The most alkaline forming are: fig juice, green juices of all green vegetables and tops, carrot, beet, celery, pineapple and citrus juices."

Eating too much protein from industrial meat, consuming processed dairy and products, eating high levels of sugar, and consuming white flour and hydrogenated oils for long periods of time keeps you on the acidic side of this equation, and simply overwhelms your immune system. Of course, the stress of modern life and the general dysfunctions of our modern world are important psychological factors in allowing cancer to grow in your body.

Even modern medicine can contribute to us being vulnerable to cancer, by prescribing antibiotics to kill bugs or prevent infection when we undergo medical procedures. Unfortunately, there is a well-documented increased incidence of cancer among people who take antibiotics frequently. Among women who are heavy users of antibiotics, good studies show the risk of breast cancer doubles. Possibly this occurs because the antibiotics kill off the beneficial bacteria in your intestines and allow a period of time in which cancer cells could thrive (or migrate), because your protective flora and fauna have been killed off by the antibiotics.

Every time you take antibiotics, make sure you err on the side of caution and take a dose of beneficial, pro-biotic, acidophilus live bacteria cultures. Look for these products in the refrigerated section of your local health food store. The yoghurt you buy in the supermarket does not qualify, as the manufacturers pasteurize the products and kill off all live cultures. Natural yoghurts from the health food store, including a product called Bio-K that comes refrigerated in small, portion sized bottles, help restore the natural flora and fauna of beneficial bacteria in your intestinal tract. Work with them—so they can work for you.

An Anti-Cancer Diet

In the beginning of this chapter, I mentioned that primitive peoples all over the world had no heart disease or cancer. I suggest you eat like them to be truly healthy. Dr. Weston A. Price, the pioneering dentist from Cleveland, Ohio, who traveled the world researching the diets of these primitive peoples in the 1920s and 1930s ,was the first to describe the common elements in the diet between healthy South Sea Islanders, Native Americans, Africans, and Eskimos.

Here's the heart healthy, anti-cancer diet of the world's healthiest peoples:

AN ANTI CANCER DIET
Don't eat refined or denatured foods such as sugar or corn syrup, white flour, canned foods, pasteurized homogenized, skim or low-fat milk; refined or hydrogenated vegetable oils; artificial vitamins or toxic additives and colorings, or protein powders. Never use polyunsaturated vegetable oils.
Never eat powdered eggs, powdered milk or foods that contain them. Most diary products in America contain powdered milk. It's an "industry standard" practice and they aren't required to put it on the label.

Eat animal proteins and fat from fish and other seafood, water and land fowl, land animals, eggs, whole milk, whole milk products, reptiles and insects.

Eat some animal products raw. Meats and fish are safe to eat raw as long as they've been frozen for 14 days and thawed out. Both primitive and traditional native diets contain high enzyme foods such as raw dairy products (milks or cheeses that aren't pasteurized or homogenized), raw meat or fish, raw honey, wine and unpasteurized beer, naturally preserved lacto-fermented vegetables, fresh fruit juice, and fruits.

Eat whole, natural foods. Eat only foods that will spoil—but eat them before they do.

Prepare homemade meat stocks and broths from the bones of chicken, beef, lamb or fish and use in sauces and stews. Freeze them and use as needed.

Use fresh whole grains and nuts that have been prepared by soaking, sprouting or sour leavening to neutralize phytic acid and other anti-nutrients.

Use natural sea salts. I use Real Salt, an ancient sea bed salt from southern Utah.

Eat only natural sweeteners, such as honey, maple syrup, brown rice sugar, honey comb, etc.

Eat naturally raised, organic, meat including fish, seafood, poultry, buffalo, beef, lamb, game, organ meats, and eggs.

Eat whole, naturally produced milk products from pasture fed cows, preferably raw and fermented, such as whole yoghurt, cultured butter, whole cheeses and fresh and sour cream.

Use only traditional fats and oils including butter and other animal fats, extra virgin olive oil, expeller pressed sesame and flax oil, and the tropical oils from coconut and palm.

Eat as much fruit as you can.

Eat fresh vegetables, preferably organic, in salads and soups, or lightly steamed.

A Final Note on Science and Spirit

When I was almost finished writing this book, I had the good fortune of having it read by a doctor who had practiced medicine in

Santa Barbara since 1963. Needless to say, I was pleased an M.D. liked my book and was strongly supportive of my efforts. We had a great lunch together at Via Maestra, an excellent Italian deli in the San Roque district of Santa Barbara, and the good doctor's story had a surprising twist that needs to be included here.

I should add first that I tried hard to leave the spiritual side of health out of *The Santa Barbara Diet*, because I wanted this book to be science-based. By writing it, I wanted to help millions of people understand what it takes to be healthy and felt having my book backed by research would be the best way. Because so many books have been written telling you how important your attitude is—in both creating and healing cancer—I thought I'd stick with the science side of the equation and leave out the spiritual side.

So I was surprised when the doctor asked me what I thought of the spiritual side of healing, and why I'd left it out. I explained why I'd left it out, and a little while later, between bites of delicious pumpkin ravioli, I asked him the magic question: *Have you ever had any patients who've healed or cured themselves of cancer?*

He told me that over the years he'd had half a dozen individuals, both men and women, with a terminal prognosis, "usually six months to live or less," who had healed their cancer and caused it to go into total remission. All of them, he asserted, had one thing in common—a strong desire to live and the willingness to be their own best advocate. This attitude went hand in hand with them accepting personal responsibility for their treatment and the care of their own body.

As patients, they used the tools of modern medicine to varying degrees, yet they all had a common thread of believing in their body's strength and power to heal itself. All of them were willing to do whatever it took to rid their body of cancer. Perhaps, the most unusual of them was a man who, when told he had prostate cancer and wouldn't have long to live, replied that he knew *exactly* what to do. When the doctor inquired what he meant, he said, "You eat a can of asparagus every day and drink all the juice in the can. That's what makes it go away...."

Was there something in that patient's genetic make-up that made this treatment work for him? Or was it his faith that if he ate the asparagus, his cancer *would* go away? Neither the doctor nor I had a clue what healed him, but a year later when he had his final check-up, all traces of cancer had vanished from his body.

He continued to tell me that once on the same day, he'd given two women patients the same prognosis for colon cancer. "You should get your affairs in order, because the odds are very high, you have less than six months to live," he advised them. The first woman was in an abusive relationship with her husband who was an alcoholic and a person the doctor knew quite well. He advised her to think seriously about leaving her husband, and she responded, "I can't." Within three months, she was dead.

The other woman, diagnosed with colon cancer and given a prognosis of a short time to live, took a different path. She'd been advised by a surgeon to have at least one foot of her cancerous colon removed, and she said, "Absolutely not." Her initial reaction to the doctor's prognosis was to say, "I'm not going to die in six months—I'm going to live for another ten years—or more...." This patient was an older woman who had never been married and had come to Santa Barbara after growing up in a large town on the Eastern seaboard. She started researching what treatments she would need and began to work on healing herself. Her treatment of choice was a mix of meditation, vitamins, healthy living, and relatively non-invasive medical treatments for cancer. Over ten years later, after she had died, the doctor did an autopsy and took along the surgeon who had wanted to operate on her colon. With the autopsy, both of them could clearly see she had died of natural causes and didn't have any traces of colon cancer in her body at the time of death.

The biggest surprise of all came at our lunch meeting when the doctor continued his story by telling me of his own recovery from cancer. Like so many other doctors, after taking over the practice of another doctor, he'd become a workaholic. But that ended for him when he started becoming very ill. After an unexplained weight loss of 30 pounds, he got a scan of his pancreas, revealing the dark, tell-tale sign of a large tumor. He knew it was time for a change in his life, so he settled his affairs and moved to Kaua'i in the Hawaiian Islands—either to die or to get well.

In talking about it over our good Italian food on a sunny afternoon, he said that he knew in the core of his being—in his heart of hearts—what he had to do. He said, "You have to strip everything else away and get down to the core of your being. You have to answer the questions for yourself of why you're here, what you want to accomplish, and why you want to keep living. You have to dig down deep into your own personal center of knowingness—and discover what you should do to heal yourself...."

In Kaua'i, he meditated on these questions and found the strength to answer them. He started out swimming in the ocean—he could only do a little bit at first—and then more, and then built up to doing long ocean swims. His path of healing was to let the healing forces of the sun and the water connect him to the spirit that moves in all things. And most of all—listening to his body—and eating whatever his spirit compelled him to eat. Gradually, he healed himself....

Thirteen years later, we sat in the sunlight eating excellent food, and I felt my doctor friend's story was one I should share with you. Obviously, healing and surviving some of the obstacles life hurls your way involves both science and spirit. I'm thankful to the good doctor for his help in reviewing my manuscript—and also for sharing his remarkable story.

After hearing his story, I went and re-read one of the first books on self-healing from a terminal disease, *Anatomy of an Illness*, by Norman Cousins published in 1976. One of the little noticed practices that Norman Cousins did to heal himself was taking 25,000 milligrams daily of vitamin C intravenously. As I mentioned in the chapter on vitamin C, if you're ill, you need to take vitamin C to the limits of your bowel tolerance. Cousin's book has been often cited by health authors, and they mention he cured himself by using the power of laughter—but they usually neglect to mention he also used high doses of vitamin C.

Norman Cousins also quoted Russian author Boris Pasternak from his novel, *Dr. Zhivago*, as saying, "Your health is bound to be affected, if, day after day, you say the opposite of what you feel, if you grovel before what you dislike, and rejoice at what brings you nothing but misfortune. Our nervous system isn't just a fiction; it's a part of our physical body, and our soul exists in space, and is inside us, like the teeth in our mouth. It can't be forever violated with impunity."

No one can deny there can be a powerful emotional component of cancer and of terminal disease. To heal yourself you need to clear your emotions and get down to the very center of your *knowingness*.

There is truth in what Albert Schweitzer observed in the jungles of Africa in the early years of this century, and wrote about in his book, *Out of My Life and Thought*: "The witch doctor succeeds for the same reason all of us succeed. Each patient carries his own doctor inside of him. They come to us not knowing that truth. We are at our best when we give the doctor who resides within each patient a chance to go to work."

And don't forget to take your vitamin C!

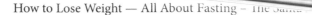

CHAPTER NINE

How To Lose Weight—
All About Fasting

Do diets work? Of course they don't! How many times have you tried to lose weight with a diet plan, lost a little, and then gained it all right back again? This is the pattern that's all too familiar to the millions of Americans who go on diets to lose weight every year.

Other than looking around your local shopping mall or food store and checking out the expanding girth of our fellow Americans, the best proof of the failure of diets is a quick visit to your local used book store. Find any diet books there? The reason there aren't more diet books on the shelves is because sellers know the used ones don't sell—everyone knows diets don't work. Yet hope springs eternal, and there's always a new crop of diet books that pop up for people to try again.

The Santa Barbara Diet is different than any other book published about diet. It's an A-Z, "how-to" guide for good health, not your typical diet book promoted by a New York publisher, ghost written by a professional author, featuring the front man (the author!) with the letters PhD or MD after his name. I've figured out what you and I need to do for our good health, and I've let the chips fall where they may in telling the story. If I happen to offend Donald Rumsfield, Michael Milliken, the Monsanto Corporation, or Dean Foods, all I can say is—*too bad!*

Probably the single greatest reason you and I can't stay on diets is that cutting back on calories makes us very hungry. Being typical Americans, we start doing everything at once and we want quick results. We start working out more, then try to cut back on our eating at the same time. This doesn't work! It makes us hungry and we go off the diet.

If you're like most people, you've gained about one pound each year since high school. When I started trying to lose weight, this is exactly where I found myself. Do the math, and find out for yourself. What is really surprising and rarely noticed is how your body manages to only gain about one pound each year, despite all the extra calories you take in. This is, of course, the traditional amount of weight gain, but today there are many people in America gaining much more than one pound each year. Why is this?

The Lethal Combo

Probably the biggest factor in weight gain is the dietary double whammy of half your sugar consumption coming from high fructose corn syrup combined with the toxic effects of eating hydrogenated soybean oils. It's been well documented in both test rats and humans that high fructose corn syrup causes quicker weight gain than even sugar's empty calories. And close to 80% of the oil consumed in the United States is vegetable oil—mostly soy or cheap cottonseed oils— and all of them are partially or fully hydrogenated to prevent rancidity. Eating soy oil is a hazard to your health, as it contains *goitrogens*— plant hormones, such as soy isoflavones—that affect your thyroid and slow down your metabolism.

We currently feed large amounts of processed soy products to animals here in America, and the reason why livestock producers use so much soy is that it causes quick weight gain. Advantageous, of course, if you're raising livestock—but if you're trying to lose weight—not so good!

Think you don't eat oil from soybeans? Look around your refrigerator—ketchup, mayonnaise, salad dressing, mustard, margarine—everything in your refrigerator has soybean oil in it. Not to mention the obvious products containing soy oil, like potato chips, snacks foods, candy bars, cookies, etc.

Because the FDA required labeling of trans fats in 2006, soybean producers are rushing new soybeans to market that are engineered to have low levels of *linolenic acid*, an alteration that allows them to be crushed without needing hydrogenation. It's a fact that the current crops of hydrogenated soybean oil and other products made from the oil have a shelf life of *from here to eternity*. Would you believe me if I told you most bugs and insects are too smart to eat hydrogenated soybean oil products? Do a little science experiment for yourself: Put a dish of butter out in your garden and put out a dish of cheap margarine or Crisco. Which one do the ants, wasps, and bees favor? Any guess which one might be better for you or more nutritious?

In Asia, the traditional use for crushed soybean oil was to burn it in lamps, to make soap, to grease axles, and lubricate machinery. Soybeans were first cultivated in China, but the Chinese never consumed them, unless they were very poor and couldn't obtain anything else. The preferred oils in China have always been lard (pig fat), sesame oil, peanut oil, and rapeseed oil. Could this have something to do with the extremely low rates of heart disease and breast cancer in China?

One of the most important factors, I believe, in low rates of these diseases in China is their very low consumption of polyunsaturated vegetable oils and toxic hydrogenated oils, such as margarine, Better Than Butter, and Crisco. Another factor is that by living much further down the food chain and not eating food products made by American agri-business, the Chinese get a lot more vitamins and minerals in their diet. Also, they've been were lucky enough to never be exposed to the dietary and medical experts here in America who have recommended for the last 70 years that you consume allegedly "heart healthy" polyunsaturated vegetable oils—like so many Americans did. As mentioned earlier, the Chinese also have much less exposure to synthetic chemical hormones and antibiotics in their diet than American consumers.

One of the biggest surprises I got in researching this book was finding out just how wrong the dietary advice is that we are given by our so-called medical authorities. The closest parallel I can think of to my discoveries about false nutritional advice is the many lies our government dished out back in the '60s and '70s in regards to "winning" the war in Vietnam. Much of the advice America's dietary experts is now giving you is as deeply flawed as the premise for going to war in Vietnam—and now Iraq.

As I write this, America is deeply enmeshed in another losing war in Iraq, repeating the same brutal folly of America's intervention into a civil war in Vietnam. Once you realize that so many of the verities trotted out by the experts are either partially or completely wrong, *you realize you need to start thinking for yourself*—in matters political as well as dietary and health.

Given the untruths fostered on us by our American food manufacturing business and the government that supports it, here is some basic advice about losing weight that most diet books won't give you:

- ✓ **Don't eat products with high fructose corn syrup.**
- ✓ **Don't eat foods containing soy or vegetable oils.** Stay away from all polyunsaturated oils.
- ✓ **Only eat natural sugars, such as honey, maple syrup, brown rice syrup, stevia, agave syrup, etc.** Avoid eating anything but small amounts of sucrose (sugar).
- ✓ **Eat coconut or olive oils.** Coconut oils are medium chain fatty acids that stimulate your metabolism and cause you to lose weight. Olive oil is simply high quality oil that's good for you. Eat fat to lose fat—it sounds counter-intuitive, but it works. It's also easier to lose weight when you're not craving fats or sugars. Eating high quality saturated fats is the key to ending sugar cravings.

Key to Healthy Weight Loss

When it comes to losing weight, absolutely nothing works better than fasting. Fasting is simply the most amazing way to diet you've ever encountered. Once you learn how to fast, you'll find it melts pounds off by burning fat at an amazing pace. Typically, you'll lose one to two pounds each day. How's that for dieting? And once you get through the first 48 hours—you won't feel hungry again. That's right—NO HUNGER.

When it comes to dieting, I originally started out recommending a fasting routine, but soon realized it was irresponsible of me to tell Americans to fast. I had to modify my fasting recommendations to include nutritional supplements.

What caused me to change recommending a traditional fasting program was reading articles about dieters having problems with thinning hair or even severe hair loss. The cause of this? Most

American's are on the razor's edge of malnutrition, and losing hair is a sure sign of this. It might sound odd to say someone who is obese is malnourished, but it's true.

I've dealt with this diet problem by developing what I call *nutritionally assisted fasting*—the key to healthy fasting. You go on a fast, but you take vitamin and mineral supplements to ensure you're not going to have hair thinning or loss. Surprisingly enough, the supplements I'm recommending might actually make your hair grow thicker.

The reason dieters have hair loss is an obvious proof of just how deficient in essential vitamins and minerals we Americans are. It's a fact that American soils have been strip-mined of nutrients for the last 100 years, and most foods in this country are grown with fertilizers made from petroleum by-products. In America, our foods look good, but are nutritionally deficient.

You'll find this out for yourself when you start adequately supplementing your diet with the vitamins, minerals and supplements I'm recommending. Be patient when you first start taking vitamins, minerals and nutritional oils—sometimes it takes as much as one to six months before the effects kick in.

You may be thinking you're healthy, and I thought I was healthy, too, but I kept feeling better and better as the cumulative effect of my nutritional program increased. It took almost three months of taking cod liver oil, magnesium, coconut oil, wheat germ oil, brewer's yeast and high doses of vitamin C before the full benefits were realized. A lot of the fatigue and overall all malaise I'd attributed to aging turned out to be the cumulative effects of years of vitamin and mineral deficiencies. If your primary diet is fresh foods grown in rich organic soil, you probably won't have any problems fasting to lose weight. But if this is your diet, you're certainly not the average American!

Fasting and Your Liver

The reason why fasting works so well is our bodies have thousands of years of genetic programming designed to help us go long periods of time without eating. It's very likely a large amount of the benefits of fasting primarily come from giving your liver and digestive system a breathing spell, in which they turn from digesting foods to cleaning house on your system.

When it comes to caring for your body, fasting is the single most important thing you will ever do for your liver. You can't live very long without your liver functioning, and taking care of it is essential to your good health.

As important as your liver is to your daily life, it's surprising how little thought we give to its many complicated functions. Your liver is your largest internal organ, weighing almost three pounds. Because it's so essential for life, your liver is designed for massive redundancy, with two separate lobes operating independently of each other. Amazingly enough, each separate unit is composed of about 50,000 small lobules that function like individual, smaller livers. Your brain is the only other organ whose design is as complex and multi-faceted as your liver.

Because of your liver's many functions in processing, converting, distributing, and storing your body's fuel supply, your very life itself depends upon your liver. It's the primary organ in converting food into the living energy that sustains your body. Yet most of us go through our daily lives paying little attention to this miraculous organ that filters about one and a half quarts of blood every minute.

Your liver is so essential, it's the only organ in your body that can regenerate itself after a portion is removed. After a loss of up to 75% of the liver, due to injury or surgery, the remaining liver can grow back and be restored to normal size within a few months. No one has ever devised an artificial liver, because its many functions would be so hard to replicate. In addition to producing hormones and storing nutrients, your liver disassembles the proteins you eat and converts them into amino acids.

When it comes to fasting, the most important function to support is the job of filtering and purifying your blood. As blood enters our liver, specialized immune cells called *phagocytes* remove and destroy bacteria and other foreign matter. Acting together with the phagocytes are specialized cells called *hepatocytes* that manufacture specialized enzymes for any and every new waste product or toxin that enters the liver. This is one of the many miracles your liver does every minute of the day.

The ability of these special hepatocytes to design and manufacture new enzymes to deal with new chemicals or toxins encountered and also treat excess hormone levels of estrogen, cortisol, and adrenaline, is nothing short of the miraculous. Researchers can only marvel at the fact that hepatocytes will, on demand, fabricate the specific enzyme needed to metabolize a specific toxin.

Everything you take into your body gets filtered through your liver, including toxic by-products of poor food choices, alcohol, tobacco, chemicals, pesticides, caffeine, and the residues of prescription drugs. While the liver does an excellent job of handling those substances, some of the products that can overload the liver's cleansing capacity are anabolic steroids, oral contraceptives, high dose acetaminophen (Tylenol), aspirin, and drugs used in chemotherapy. Herbs that have stimulating, energizing and revitalizing properties for your liver are rosemary, garlic, dandelion root, black Cohosh, gentian, and cascara sagrada.

Despite the many news reports you've read of scientific studies showing how small amounts of alcohol, usually wine, are good for you, your liver puts the lie to those studies. Alcohol is not good for your liver. At least 10% of the calories ingested in America are alcohol, so I'd be remiss in not saying that alcohol, even in moderate quantities, *can damage your liver*. For occasional drinkers, the damage is temporary, and the liver can usually bounce back after several days of rest and clean living. But more often, those who drink heavily never give their liver a chance to recuperate, and such drinking can cause serious liver damage.

Cirrhosis of the liver is a condition in which the liver damaged by disease or alcohol grows back (regenerates) but doesn't grow back properly. The regenerated liver tissue is rough, covered with fibrous scar tissue and lumpy irregular nodules. If no rest cycles or care are given, eventually the liver becomes so scarred by cirrhosis, it can't do its work, and the afflicted person dies of liver failure.

One of the reasons why fasting works so well is that it gives your liver a rest from digesting food and lets it go to work cleaning up toxins in your body. In addition to burning up your fat as fuel (one gram of fat contains more than twice as much energy as one gram of carbohydrate), your liver turns to burning up bacteria, viruses, fibroid tumors, and stored pollutants as fuel sources.

Your liver is busy trying to take care of your health in these modern times, so it's always working overtime. The Environmental Protection Agency has identified over 65,000 toxic chemicals used in the U.S. each year, and traces of some of them are in our food. Agriculture alone releases over one billion pounds of highly toxic pesticides each year, and residues of them end up in our bodies.

When your body is overloaded with toxins, those toxins can overload your lymph system as well as your liver, and end up being stored in fat and muscle tissue. Fasting is, of course, a general tune-up for your lymph system. Obviously, a healthy, high functioning liver and lymph system are essential for your good health. The reason why I've given you this small primer on your liver is because it's the organ that will burn up your fat supplies when you fast, helping you to lose weight.

Fasting: The Ultimate Fat Burner

Fat is what we're interested in getting rid of, and fasting is the best way to get rid of fat. Fat is an excellent fuel for your metabolism, the single most efficient stored fuel in your body, providing almost 3,500 calories per pound. That's why fat is so hard to get rid of with conventional diets. It takes a lot of exercise to burn up a pound of fat.

The reason why our bodies are so efficient at storing fat can be found in our genetic heritage. Our genes are almost identical to those of our earliest common ancestors who lived 40,000 or more years ago. Those ancestors' genes were programmed to survive periods when little food was available by making them very efficient at storing food during times of plenty. Those whose bodies evolved to store fat efficiently survived, reproduced, and passed this capability to their descendants.

The legacy of this feast and famine lifestyle of our early ancestors is something scientists call our "thrifty gene," which is your genetic predisposition to hoard fat in preparation for the next famine. This hoarding creates a strong tendency for you to have higher than normal levels of insulin in your blood in times of plenty, a condition that greatly increases the storage capacity of your body's fat cells. Your body wants to store fats whenever it can to provide for times of potential food shortage, such as late winter or early spring, when food might not be available in a hunter/gatherer society.

Our primitive ancestors, in addition to developing the capacity to store fat, also developed the capacity to go for long periods of time without eating. You're programmed this way because your ancestors needed the capability to metabolize your body's supplies of fat and use it as fuel. Our ancestors had to have this capability, because they often had to survive the lack of food during drought conditions or changing patterns of animal migration.

Surprisingly enough, your body also is designed to function at a high level and can go without food for 7 to 10 days or even as long as 30 days. When you fast, you find yourself sleeping less, mentally alert, and able to perform at a high level. This is exactly the sort of condition you'd want to be in if it was a matter of survival for you to hunt down a wild animal to bring food home for the hungry members of your tribe.

What to Expect While Fasting

Probably the most dramatic changes that occur during fasting take place in the first three days, as your body switches from burning glucose (blood sugar), stored in your liver as *glycogen*, to burning fat. There is usually enough glycogen stored in your liver to fuel your body for 8 to 12 hours, becoming depleted within 24 hours when your body switches over to *ketosis*.

Ketosis, or ketone production, is the burning of fatty acids as fuel instead of glucose. This shift from sugar burning to fat burning usually occurs on the second day of fasting and is finished by the third day. In this interim period, there isn't glucose available, and the energy from fat conversion isn't enough to supply your body's fuel needs yet. Your body then converts *glycerol*, available in your fat stores, to glucose.

But this still isn't enough fuel for the body to run. Your body makes up the difference by breaking down proteins from muscle tissue and burning them up in your liver to make glucose. Typically, your body uses 60 to 84 grams of protein on the second day (about two to three ounces of muscle tissue). By the third day, ketone production is sufficient to fuel your body from your fat supplies, and only very tiny amounts of muscle tissue are used to run your body.

Misunderstanding this process is where the myth comes from that fasting makes you lose muscle. Nothing could be further from the truth. Your body is designed to run on your fat supplies for as long as 30 days without much of a problem. Your body has a long evolutionary history of being designed to protect muscle tissue—of which most major organs, including your heart, are composed of. Your fat cells are the first to go, while the muscle stays.

Concerns have been raised by some medical practitioners that fasting can cause muscle loss resulting from the ketosis state into which the body is put by fasting. Often this concern comes from confusion between *ketoacidosis* and *ketosis*. The two processes have similarities but are very different in nature. Ketoacidosis occurs when ketone levels rise sharply because of an abnormal physical state that can occur in type I diabetics or alcoholics. Fasting doesn't cause ketoacidosis.

Ketosis, which does occur during fasting, happens when ketone bodies in the blood rise higher than normal levels of (0.2 mmol/l), yet stay well below the high levels associated with ketoacidosis. Your body has normal, healthy biochemical mechanisms to regulate ketosis, both how long it lasts and to balance it out. Your kidneys play a key role in ketosis by analyzing the high levels of ketone acids in your blood and excreting ammonia to balance acid/base levels and prevent ketoacidosis.

This balancing job of your kidneys also protects the body from the loss of large quantities of potassium and sodium in urine during fasting. On the second day of fasting before the shift to ketosis, you excrete significant amounts of potassium and sodium. Once your body begins burning fat for fuel, your kidneys help to regulate your body's electrolyte balance and conserve sodium and potassium.

Fasting Benefits and Precautions

Obviously, giving your liver the time to rejuvenate itself and do some house cleaning on your immune system is a powerful benefit from fasting. But it's truly surprising that so many other medical conditions can be helped or even cured by fasting. In 1988, a clinical trial of 88 people with acute pancreatitis showed fasting to work better than any other medical treatment, as reported in a helpful book by Stephen Buhner, *The Fasting Path: The Way to Spiritual, Physical and Emotional Enlightenment*. Fasting is also extremely beneficial to those with chronic cardiovascular disease or congestive heart failure. Fasting increases HDL cholesterol levels and lowers triglycerides, blood pressure, and total cholesterol. A number of studies have shown that fasting is effective in treating both osteoarthritis and rheumatoid arthritis. Because of its long term effects on metabolism and how fat is stored in your body, fasting is also effective in treating type II diabetes.

The beauty of fasting to lose weight is that the fatter you are, the more fat is converted to fuel each day. Most people lose one to two pounds each day when they fast. But a word to the wise—you should never confuse fasting with starvation. Starvation is what occurs when your body has exhausted its stores of fat and begins to burn the protein in muscle tissue for fuel. When you look at what your body is composed of, it isn't hard to see that you have plenty of fat to burn.

THE HUMAN BODY
.5 to 1% Sugars
1 to 2% Vitamins and minerals
7% Protein
20% Fat
70% Water

I should mention here that the kind of fasting practiced during the Islamic holiday, Ramadan, is not the kind of fasting I'm talking about, nor the sort of traditional fasting practiced throughout the centuries. The current Islamic practice is to go all day without drinking water or eating, then gather with family and friends and eat a big meal in the evening. It's not the kind of fasting I'm recommending. Always drink large amounts of water when you fast; it helps your body cleanse itself and helps your liver and kidneys with the process of ketosis. I usually drink at least two quarts a day of water when I fast.

Fasting Stories

How long can humans fast? The longest fast I've heard of was done by sixties comedian Dick Gregory, who once fasted for 81 days.

Gregory, who later became known as a humanitarian and social activist, at one time weighed almost 350 pounds, smoked four packs of cigarettes daily, and downed a quart of scotch each day. After becoming a fasting and fitness addict, he ran in eight Boston Marathons. In 1976, for the Bi-Centennial Celebration, he ran from Los Angeles to New York, a total of 2,980 miles, drinking only fruit and vegetable juices. Dick's autobiography, *NIGGER*, has sold over seven million copies.

A different sort of fasting than Dick Gregory did was the involuntary fast by Ralph Flores and Helen Klaben when their plane crashed in a remote area of British Columbia in 1963. They had only melted snow to drink and a few biscuits to live on for 49 days until they were rescued. They were in excellent shape when they were rescued, but Ralph had lost 51 pounds and Helen lost 45 pounds. Ms. Klaben later said she'd been contemplating going on a diet, but a "plane crash diet" wasn't exactly what she'd had in mind.

Another fasting account was written by health pioneer and originator of health food stores, Paul C. Bragg, of Santa Barbara, California. Here is an excerpt from his book, *The Miracle of Fasting*, about going to India to meet Mahatma Gandhi, reprinted here by permission:

> *The date I met Gandhi was July 27, 1946, in New Delhi, which would become the capital of the New Republic of India a year and a month later. At Gandhi's headquarters there, I received permission to accompany this amazing man on a 21 day fasting trip eastward through India's villages, where he would walk with the people and help them with their problems. At that time, the average Indian earned about ten cents a day and starvation was a way of life. To show he shared their plight, this saintly and compassionate spiritual leader was planning to travel on foot, without food, only water for three weeks. Gandhi was 77 years of age and looked very frail in appearance. But his looks were indeed deceiving! This man was as tower of strength, physically, mentally and*

spiritually. His stamina, endurance, energy and mental abilities were astounding to everyone!

The trek began at sun up. The heat and humidity were the worst I have ever experienced. I have spent time in some of the hottest spots in the world, including Death Valley in California, the Sahara Desert and across North America on an 800 mile bicycle trip in intense summer heat. But never once did Gandhi seem to tire. Never once did he falter in his brisk pace of walking. The only time he sat down was during talks with the villagers. He would speak for 20 minutes, and then answer questions for 20 minutes. Then we continued down the hot, dusty road to the next village. Gandhi ate nothing and drank only water flavored with lemon and honey.

Many who tried to travel with him fell by the wayside, suffering from heat and exhaustion. But Gandhi was inexhaustible. I have been an athlete and a hiker all my life, but I have never seen anyone who had the physical stamina and energy that Gandhi had. Each day he walked and talked until sundown before stopping for a rest. During the 21 day fasting walk, I had many talks with Gandhi on the power of fasting. Of all I learned from him, this statement by him seems to me the summation: "All the vitality and energy I have comes to me because my body is purified by fasting."

Walking mile after mile from village to village, he gave the people courage and hope that a better life was coming to them.

*His internal strength and beautiful pure soul
were so powerful that weak people felt strong
after seeing him and hearing his brilliant
wisdom. He gave his unlimited strength to the
discouraged and the sick. He brought bright
light and love where there was darkness.
Gandhi told the people to fast and purify
their bodies and they would find peace and
joy on earth. Gandhi said, "The light of the
world will illuminate within you, when you
fast and purify yourself."*

*The trip with Gandhi is an experience
I will never forget! This physically small
man was a spiritual giant. He led millions
of people to independence from the mighty
British Empire without striking a single
physical blow. Yet with all his power and
influence, he was completely without
arrogance. Characteristically, on the day of
India's independence, Gandhi took no part in
the celebrations that went on all over India;
instead he spent the day in fasting and prayer
in his garden.*

The Spiritual Power of Fasting

The idea of going without food for two to ten days might seem crazy to the average American, but there's good reasons why fasting is the oldest medical treatment known. As well as the medical reasons for fasting, there's a powerful spiritual component to fasting too. It isn't an accident that the Bible refers to fasting 74 times. If you're a Christian and you fast, you're in good company as Moses, Elijah, and Jesus all fasted. In other religious and philosophical traditions, some of those who advocated fasting are Mohammed, Buddha, Hippocrates, Plato, Plutarch, Pythagoras, and Socrates. The Native American spiritual tradition here in America has long used fasting as a method for individuals to seek wisdom and spirituality through their own personal vision quest. It is, of course, mildly sacreligious to speak of the time honored practice of fasting as only a diet program.

Fasting is a powerful, energy filled, transforming experience that will connect you to the spiritual side of life so often ignored in our modern, materialistic world. Often, the practice of denying yourself food opens your psychic floodgates to memories, dreams, and even visions that come to you when you do something as simple as stopping eating for a few days.

On a recent fast, I suddenly woke in the middle of the night and thought of the dream I'd been having: I was five or six years old and sitting up on my bed in a room in Madison, Wisconsin. Sunlight was streaming through the trees outside, the leaves were budding out, and everything was colored a bright and beautiful green. Green of early summer, green of new leaves; insects were buzzing, birds were singing, and I could feel the living pulse of the earth. I started tingling with excitement at what the day might bring. When was the last time you felt like that?

For the first two days of a fast, you might find yourself up at night looking at cookbooks and obsessing over food. It's a good time to deal with your various food addictions, meditate upon them and figure out how you're going to overcome them. You need to develop the consciousness to be the master of your habits instead of a servant to your addictions. Fasting will take you there!

Another time during a fast, I suddenly remembered a childhood memory of being lost somewhere in the fields of Wisconsin and taking half an hour to eat a Milky Way candy bar. Lying on my back on a Huckleberry Finn sort of afternoon with the clouds streaming by, day dreaming and eating that candy bar, one tiny nibble at a time. That's the sort of food enjoyment fasting helps you to develop, making you slow down and appreciate your food.

I'm not a purist about caffeine during fasts. Of course, it's better to go without coffee, but if you're hooked on the stuff like most Americans, I'd rather see you succeed at a fast than break if off because of your caffeine addiction. If decaf works for you, that would be a healthier alternative while fasting.

Get Started

I've had the most success with fasting by using a mixture of water, maple syrup, and lemon juice. You can drink all you want of this mixture while you fast and it will help your body purify itself. The maple syrup helps balance out your glucose levels and gives your brain fuel. Your brain runs on glucose and this mixture works well at getting you through the critical first two days of a fast.

You also want to take a multiple vitamin, cod liver oil, wheat germ oil, coconut oil, magnesium, and brewer's yeast to make sure you're not lacking in essential nutrients.

NUTRITIONAL SUPPLEMENTS TO TAKE WHILE FASTING
1 TBSP of coconut oil. Warm slightly to drink it or add to hot herbal tea (120 calories). Use as much as 6 TBSP if needed. Coconut oil is a high quality, saturated fat that stimulates your metabolism and causes you to lose weight.
1 TSP of wheat germ oil or pumpkin seed oil. (40 calories.)
1 TSP of cod liver oil. (40 calories)
1 TBSP of brewer's yeast. Buy in bulk at your local health food store. This is what prevents hair loss while dieting. Brewer's yeast is in almost all pet foods or livestock feeds sold, and is why it says on the side of the bag: "For a shiny coat or glossy fur." It's loaded with B vitamins and will make your hair grow.
One dose of a good multiple vitamin and mineral combination.
250 to 500 milligrams of magnesium. It's estimated as many as 80% of all Americans are deficient in this mineral that is absolutely essential for your heart functions. If you have kidney disease, consult your doctor before taking magnesium supplements.
8 ounces of fresh squeezed orange juice. (120 Calories) Use any type of fresh squeezed juice, or frozen if you have to. Make sure you only use 100% juice. I pour out one inch of juice, add vitamin C crystals and brewers yeast and drink it down. Then I enjoy the rest of the juice. Carrot juice is also a good alternative to orange juice.

If you drink two quarts daily of this maple syrup mix and take the supplements, you will be consuming about 600 calories. This is similar to the amount of calories you're allowed in hospital-supervised weight loss programs, where they sell you daily meals that cost $10 to $20 per day.

Here's how to do it: Take a one gallon jar, fill it half full of good water, add 6 tablespoons of freshly squeezed lemon juice and six tablespoons of maple syrup and mix well. Adjust the proportions according to your own needs. Sprinkle in some cayenne pepper (optional), and continue filling with cold water. This is what you're going to run your body on for the next (X) days.

You're the one who has to fill in that last blank! If it's your first fast, going for three or five days is plenty. I routinely fast for seven to ten days without much trouble. Once you learn how to fast, you've gained an incredible skill for controlling your weight.

COMMON EFFECTS OF FASTING
Everyone's different, and you may experience all or none of the following effects during a fast:
Nausea. This is common and results from your body processing the toxins stored in fat. This can often be alleviated by drinking more water.
Headaches. Caffeine withdrawal usually has the most potential for causing headaches. Most headaches will pass in a few days. Drinking more water usually helps.
Body odor. This can occur from the process of eliminating toxins through your skin during a fast.
A coated tongue and bad breath. This is very common. Usually your tongue will clear to a normal healthy pink color in seven to ten days of fasting or less.
Little desire or need for sleep. You need less sleep and might even prefer to catnap more and use the extra time to get caught up on things.
Strong urine color or odor. This happens because your body is engaged in deep healing and the primary route of elimination is through the kidneys. Your urine will clear as the fast progresses.
Metallic taste in your mouth. This comes from the ketones excreted through respiration. This sensation also will pass towards the end of your fast.

The best advice for someone falling off the wagon while fasting is to eat a nourishing snack, like a can of tuna jazzed up with sun dried tomatoes, capers, fresh peppers or cilantro. Or eat fresh made hummus from sprouted garbanzo beans on lettuce leaves, or bean sprouts rolled in a wrap. Or eat an apple or a banana, have some chicken soup or broth, or some steamed vegetables; then get right back on your fast and keep going. You can do it!

I recommend taking off your clothes when you start on a fast and examining yourself closely in a mirror. Take a good look at where the fat is distributed on your body. It's also not a bad idea to keep a diary and record your weight each day. The following list of days and weights document my loss of 23 pounds by doing a nutritionally modified fast for 16 days. I started this fast at the highest weight I've ever been at in my life—225 pounds—and dropped down to 202 pounds without much effort.

DAY ONE	225 LBS.
DAY TWO	221 LBS.
DAY THREE	219 LBS.
DAY FOUR	218 LBS.
DAY FIVE	217 LBS.
DAY SIX	215 LBS.
DAY SEVEN	216 LBS.
DAY EIGHT	214 LBS.
DAY NINE	212 LBS.
DAY TEN	210 LBS.
DAY ELEVEN	208 LBS.
DAY TWELVE	206 LBS.
DAY THIRTEEN	204 LBS.
DAY FOURTEEN	204 LBS.
DAY FIFTEEN	203 LBS.
DAY SIXTEEN	202 LBS.

For those who don't think that fasting is good for you, consider these statistics showing what fasting did to my blood pressure and cholesterol levels. Because I was 54 years old and had gained a little weight, my blood pressure and cholesterol levels had started climbing:

START: January 11, 2006
Weight 225 lbs. Blood Pressure: 120 / 90
Cholesterol: TOTAL: 193
                        LDL: 124

FINISH: January 27, 2006
Weight: 202 lbs. Blood Pressure: 102 / 70
Cholesterol: TOTAL: 148
                        LDL: 82

The lemon juice and maple syrup mix is the traditional mix for fasting, but feel free to use what you have on hand, such as lime or grapefruit juice. Or use honey instead of maple syrup. I don't recommend fasting using only water, as it's much harder to do. The sugars in the maple syrup keeps your glucose levels up and help your brain function, and the citrus juice and water helps cleanse your body.

It's hard to beat maple syrup for fasting. I'm always grateful when I drink it, because I know it takes as much as 50 gallons of tree sap to cook down to one gallon of maple syrup. In the beginning, Native Americans tapped not only the maples (six species) and birches (six species), but also the butternut and hickory trees. These tree saps were used as syrups by boiling them down, but the Native Americans also drank the fresh tree sap as a tonic. There are good reasons for drinking both maple sap and syrup. They are highly nutritious foods, and one can live for weeks on maple syrup alone. Maple syrup is also known to be a good tonic and stimulant for your kidneys. It's high in calories, calcium, phosphorus, vitamin B^{12}, and it contains large amounts of iron.

Remember, if you feel nauseous or extremely tired—drink more water. Take short naps, if you need to, on the first few days. The only hard part about fasting is the first 48 hours. After that, you'll be amazed at what a tremendous fuel source your body's fat supplies are. There's nothing unnatural or unhealthy about dieting like this. Your body runs perfectly fine using fat as a fuel source.

You'll quickly realize once you learn how to fast, why it's so difficult to lose weight by the normal methods of dieting you've tried before. All exercise is good, of course, but for dieters restricting calories, fats, or sugars, exercise makes you very hungry. After all, it takes half an hour of energetic swimming to burn off 300 to 350 calories. If you did that every day for ten days, you'd metabolize only one pound of fat.

I've read that it takes 100 yards of brisk walking to burn off one M&M candy. So how can you lose weight dieting? That's why typical diets almost always fail, because it takes so much effort to get rid of fat. Very few people in an affluent, food-rich society like 21st century America have that much discipline and self control.

Fasting Help

If you feel run down or extremely tired while fasting, try the following recipe to help cleanse yourself and eliminate uric acid from your system. I call this recipe *The Swedish Broth*. It's rich in potassium and is both cleansing and nourishing. It's a good pick-me-up to help you on your fast. Use it as needed, anytime during your fast.

RECIPE FOR "SWEDISH BROTH"
1. Bring 8 cups of water to a boil.
2. Clean and slice 1½ pounds of potatoes, 1½ pounds of carrots and one leek.
3. Add to boiling water with one large bunch of parsley, one unpeeled, roughly chopped onion, garlic and herbs.
4. Cook for one hour and strain the broth.
5. Add salt and pepper, if desired, and drink the juice as a soup.
6. Add a tablespoon of high quality chicken bouillon or a tablespoon of natural miso or a cup or two of homemade turkey, chicken or beef broth, if desired.

This recipe is my own personal innovation that I've added to the ancient art and science of fasting. It's a big help on your second day, as your body switches over to burning up your fat reserves instead of your usual diet. You lose potassium and sodium during the second day and the Swedish Broth replaces it and helps you feel better. Another good practice on the second day of a fast is to drink the juice from fresh young coconuts. Like the Swedish Broth, they're high in potassium. You can usually buy them at Asian or Latin markets.

This practice of keeping potassium high helps you get through the first 48 hours, and after that—it's smooth sailing. You quickly realize your body is designed to fast. Indeed, it's part of your genetic programming to run very well on fat. Your genes aren't much different than those of salmon that swim over 3,000 miles without eating, or the gray whales that journey from Baja California to Alaska without feeding, or the polar bears that hibernate for five months and lose up to 50% of their body weight. You, too, are designed to go quite a few days without eating.

Some people worry about the lack of bowel movements during fasting, but as long as you drink plenty of fluids, you won't have any problems. If you tend to be constipated, you should mix one level tablespoon of psyllium powder with eight ounces of water or fruit juice, mix in a blender and drink quickly. Or you can use Metamucil, which is a more processed form of psyllium powder. However, avoid using any Metamucil which contains NutraSweet, Equal, or Aspartame. The last time I checked at a Wal-Mart, about 80% of the Metamucil had these toxic ingredients.

Another health aid while fasting is to rub your body thoroughly from head to toe with a natural bristle brush while you shower or bathe. This stimulates your nerve endings and improves your circulation. It also helps you get in touch with this new body you're redesigning to take with you for the rest of the journey.

When you've lost ten pounds, take off all your clothes and look at yourself in the mirror. It's simply amazing how fasting melts the fat away from your body. Your fat cells are the first to go. Now, warm some coconut oil and rub down your entire body. This is good for your skin and helps prevent stretch marks. Vitamin E or crèmes containing vitamin E can also help your skin.

After Your Fast: Keeping the Weight Off

The traditional way to end your fast is to eat four or five good ripe or canned tomatoes, add some finely chopped garlic (if desired) and heat in a pan until it almost boils. Turn off the heat and let it cool down before adding some olive oil, salt and pepper, and rice wine vinegar. Then eat lightly for a while. Eat green salads, lightly steamed vegetables, or cole slaw made from shredded cabbage, grated beets, carrots, etc. Ginger, mint, parsley, and cilantro are good additions to the cole slaw. I like to use a dressing made from honey mixed with freshly squeezed lemon, orange, lime juice, and olive oil.

The best way to keep from gaining weight back is to get your calories from eating complex carbohydrates every day. Forget that stupid advice about not eating carbs—the best way to feel full and not have food cravings is to eat *high quality complex carbohydrates*, such as brown rice, oatmeal, quinoa, soba noodles, whole wheat pasta, couscous, sweet potatoes, and barley.

Another good idea to keep weight off after you've fasted to lose excess weight is to eat an apple, a banana, and a cooked sweet potato every day for a few weeks. Surprisingly enough—this is only 360 calories. You could eat five bananas, five apples, and five cooked sweet potatoes daily and not gain weight. And those calories would be nutrient dense calories. Try eating jicama, carrots, celery, vegetables and fruit for snacks if you feel hungry. They'll fill you up and have almost no calories. Also, drinking homemade broth made from chicken, beef, or fish stock is a healthy habit of people all over the world.

You can add vegetables and other foods with this regimen—but you'll be surprised by what eating this high carb regimen does for you. Do this in addition to the vitamin and mineral program I recommended for fasting, and take one to two tablespoons of virgin coconut oil daily, also. This gives you a good nutritional base to support your continuing plan to keep weight off. The reason why I'm recommending this is because healthy primitive cultures we know of usually ate large amounts of carbohydrates. Good research has shown that people feel full and satisfied when they eat about two and a half to four pounds of food daily. The only way to do this is by eating low calorie foods that are nutrient dense.

Here's what it takes to eat 2,500 calories on a high carb regimen:

✓ 6.5 pounds of sweet potatoes
✓ 16 pounds of broccoli
✓ 9 pounds of oatmeal
✓ 9 pounds of apples

Here's what it takes to get 1,100 calories eating fast food:

✓   12 ounces of one cheeseburger and fries.

When you fast to lose weight, you run your body by burning fat, and you cut down on your body's ratio of fat to muscle. The more fat you lose, the better off you are in the long run, because muscle cells burn three times as much energy as fat cells. In other words, your fat cells are just going along for the ride! Your muscle cells, on the other hand, are doing the work of burning calories, even when you're resting or sleeping. Getting leaner is better and getting some muscles is even better.

Working out and building muscle will help you stay at the weight you want to be. This is critical to losing weight and keeping it off. I'm recommending fasting to lose weight, because it is the only way to lose weight that doesn't make you hungry all the time. Once you get close to your ideal weight—then it's time to start working out.

Remember:

✓   Muscle cells burn 13 calories per kilogram daily.
✓   Fat cells only burn 4.5 calories per kilogram daily.

I'm glad I discovered how to fast, because I certainly was a failure when it came to losing weight with any other diet I've ever tried. I've found fasting to be the best way to get control of my weight and help break the cycle of addiction to high calorie, low nutrition foods that are not only unhealthy, but put the pounds on. Now you, too, can use this amazing tool for continued health, weight loss and weight maintenance.

Here's to your success!

CHAPTER TEN

The Business Of Food: How Mass Produced Food Can Make You Sick And Fat

By now you've gotten my message that American food is all about quantity, not quality. Hopefully, you've learned how to improve your health by choosing to eat better food and get adequate amounts of vitamins and minerals. In this chapter, I'm going to take you behind the scenes of America's food industry to show you how the business of food production is at the root of our national epidemic of obesity and poor health.

We live in the land of plenty and the food on the supermarket shelves looks good enough to bear that out. But the truth is our food is often lacking in vitamins and minerals, and many common food products are toxic to your body. When it comes to agriculture, the system that has created the cheapest mass-produced foods in the world has turned a blind eye to irresponsible chemical farming methods that are beginning to have profound effects upon the health of the average American. Ever since the early 1980s, due to the corruption of the lobbying process in Washington, D.C., the interests of large agri-businesses have trumped those of people who want to eat foods complete with essential vitamins and minerals, and free of toxic chemicals.

Rapid Decline of Our Soils

America started out with some of the deepest and richest soils in the world, but after being strip mined and farmed intensively with chemical fertilizers for over 70 years, American soils are in rapid decline. Those experts who will talk about the problem believe that the widespread use of chemical fertilizers is the main culprit behind the shocking drops in vitamin and mineral contents in American foods. Adequate amounts of the chemicals nitrogen, phosphorus, and potassium ensure that crops will grow quickly, but their continued use diminishes vital nutrients in the soil.

Foods in America look good in the supermarkets, but unless they're raised organically, they can be seriously deficient in critical minerals and vitamins. The United Nations Food and Agricultural Organization concluded the use of artificial fertilizers is creating a "serious shortage" of minerals. Some studies show a 60% drop in levels of vitamins and minerals in beans since 1985, a 70% drop in potatoes, and an 80% drop in levels of nutrients in apples.

It's not just here in America, we have a problem with Industrial Farming. It's a global problem occurring wherever modern methods of agriculture are being used. In England, studies were done as far back as 1940 by R. A. McCance and E. M Widdowson to determine the nutritional content of vegetables. Their study was commissioned by England's Medical Research Council. In 1991, the same researchers were commissioned by the British Agriculture Ministry and the Royal Society of Chemistry to show the nutrient loss over the 50 year period (see Box: Nutrient Loss of Food Over 50 Years), revealing some shocking statistics, as reported in Lynn McTaggart's book, *What Doctors Don't Tell You.*

NUTRIENT LOSS OF FOOD OVER 50 YEARS	
Food:	**Nutrient Loss:**
Potatoes	35% less calcium
	45% less iron
	47% less copper
	30% less magnesium
Spring Onions	74% less calcium
Broccoli (boiled)	46% less iron
	75% less calcium
Turnip Cabbage	71% less iron
Spinach (boiled)	60% less iron
	96% less copper
Watercress	93% less copper
Carrots	48% less calcium
	75% less magnesium

Here in America, my best source of how nutritionally empty American foods are is the research done by Paul Bergner, the Director of the Rocky Mountain Center for Botanical Studies in Boulder, Colorado. He's charted the mineral content of commercial produce over the last 50 years, and his data shows levels of essential minerals and iron, manganese, and copper declining sharply. The sharpest drop he measured was iron content in lettuce which dropped from an average of 52 mg. per 100 grams to only 0.5 mg. today. He warns us that this depletion of nutrients in our food supply is leading our entire nation down the road to malnutrition and disease. He feels the lack of chromium, selenium, magnesium, and boron are beginning to cause severe health problems in America.

What got me started researching vitamin and mineral deficiencies caused by agri-business products was my discovery that the calcium and magnesium imbalance in dairy products is the primary cause of osteoporosis in America. The question is: *Why are the magnesium levels so low in dairy foods produced in America?* After all, magnesium makes up as much as 2% of the earth's crust. And with the help of bacteria in the soil, plants should naturally take up magnesium from the soil.

The problem is that the widespread use of fertilizer salts, chemicals, and herbicides have depleted soils by binding up minerals in the soil, so plants can't naturally absorb them. Modern chemical farming methods compact soils, increase salt levels, dehydrate soils, and kill the natural enzymes and bacteria in the soil. Most soils in America used for crop production are depleted of microbial life and have been saturated with chemical fertilizers and pesticides almost to the point of no return.

A good sign of soil health is the presence of earthworms, but many commonly used pesticides such as *aldicarb, carbaryl, carbofuran, benomyl,* and other soil fumigants are toxic to earthworms. Also, inorganic fertilizers, such as ammonium sulfates, acidify the soil and disrupt the life cycles and activities of resident earthworms. Many millions of acres of farmland in America are so unhealthy, they don't sustain life for earthworms. If American farming soils don't even support the needs of earthworms, how could they provide nutrition for you?

As I've said before, one of the best ways to prevent heart disease is to make sure you're getting adequate amounts of magnesium. Magnesium is absolutely essential for every beat of your heart, and it's presence in blood plasma is essential for muscle contractions. If you find yourself tired and out of breath while exercising, make sure you're getting enough magnesium. The richest foods in magnesium are organic blackstrap molasses, sunflower seeds, wheat germ, almonds, Brazil nuts, pistachios, hazelnuts, oats, pecans, brown rice, chard, barley, salmon, corn, bananas and avocados.

You need a lot of magnesium, as you only absorb about 50% of the magnesium in foods you eat. I started taking 250 milligrams and found I needed 500 milligrams daily. In America, it's an essential nutrient almost everyone is lacking.

Given the strong evidence of nutritional problems in America that are directly related to deficits of selenium, magnesium, zinc, and boron, it's hard to believe there are still medical experts, newsletter writers, and doctors saying you don't need to take supplemental vitamins, and "you get all you need" from your food. This advice comes from the same sort of doctors who say taking vitamins is a waste and only gives you *expensive urine*. Modern agri-business, of course, already has a solution to the deficiencies of vitamins and minerals in your foods. Their solution is to spray cheap synthetic chemicals, usually made from petroleum sources, onto your foods after they've been manufactured. Research shows these synthetic vitamins are poorly absorbed by your body, and they're not a good long term solution to the ongoing vitamin and mineral deficiencies in the American diet. Robert Wood, PhD., of Tufts Human Nutrition Center, has said, "only 2% of supplemental iron added to cereal is absorbed by the body." This is yet another quick-fix technological solution to an on-going problem.

These types of cheap, synthetic vitamins aren't the best solution to our country's vitamin deficiencies, but these practices have made an effect on the diseases mentioned at the end of Chapter Three, such as rickets, beriberi, goiter, and neural tube defects. The incidence of these diseases has been nearly eliminated by food manufacturers adding vitamin D, B vitamins, iodine, and folic acid to over-processed foods. That's great, but making sure you get minerals lacking in your foods by eating organic and supplementing with vitamins will help you avoid being a victim of the American epidemics of cancer, heart disease, and osteoporosis.

The Egg and You

Because the loss of nutrition is closely related, I should tell you about the vitamin and mineral deficits in one of nature's finest foods—eggs. Eggs have always been a cheap and plentiful, high quality food—unless, of course, you happen to buy them as a mass produced product in an American supermarket.

Eggs produced by standard American production methods are a food whose nutritional value is far below their potential. Coming from "farms" that are more like factories, your standard supermarket eggs are laid by chickens raised in crowded pens under artificial light, and fed sub-standard feed laced with antibiotics and growth hormones. There are over 300 million factory farm chickens in America, and almost all of them are being raised under cruel and inhumane conditions. Do your body a favor and stop eating cheap industrial eggs. Spend the extra money on the much higher quality eggs beginning to appear in our markets. Better yet, buy them from a local egg producer or raise a few chickens yourself, if you can.

Recent studies sponsored by *Mother Earth* magazine show how bad the problem is. Their tests compared eggs from free range chickens raised on pasture with eggs from industrially raised chickens. They found the free range chickens had half the cholesterol, twice the vitamin E, and four times as much beta-carotene. Additionally, the free range chickens had four times as much Omega 3 oils as the factory eggs. Their data corroborated studies done in 1988 by researcher Artemis Simopoulos that free range chickens in Greece had 13 times more Omega 3 oils than U.S. supermarket eggs. In 1973, researchers in the U.K., found eggs from free range chickens had 50% more folic acid and 70% more vitamin B12 than factory eggs. Similar results were found by Pennsylvania State University researchers in 2003 who discovered that pastured chickens had 40% more vitamin A in their yolks and twice as much vitamin E. Also, they had three times more Omega 3 oils.

A great deal of America's agriculture problems stems from the federal crop support program which encourages farmers to produce crops on the biggest possible scale they can. Federal crop supports have been a poor solution to America's chronic problem of overproduction of food. With some exceptions, American food is all about quantity—not about quality. Because of the tremendous competition in the marketplace and regulation that blatantly favors large producers, small farmers have been constantly forced off the farm.

Laws Protecting the Food Business

I realize I'm taking a certain amount of personal risk by exposing the facts of life about soy foods, processed milks and cheeses, hormone and antibiotic laden beef, vegetables and fruits lacking vitamins and minerals, and the processing methods (canning) that destroy most of the nutrients that are left. In 1991, a policy statement published in the Federal Register served notice that the FDA doesn't accept the idea that soils are depleted in any way, or that foods grown with chemicals due to modern farming methods are deficient in nutrients. The implication of this statement is the FDA would like to make it a crime for anyone to state American soils are depleted of nutrients or that dietary supplements might be needed.

As I write this, there are laws in effect in 13 states passed between 1991 and 1997, making it illegal for private citizens to give out negative information about food, unless the charge is backed up by standards defined by the law. In South Dakota, it is illegal to say generally accepted agricultural practices might make a particular food unsafe. In 1997, Texas passed the False Disparagement of Perishable Foods Products Law of 1995, which banned the dissemination of information stating a food is unsafe unless it's backed up by "reasonable and reliable scientific inquiry and facts."

Incidentally, these new laws place the burden of proving innocence upon the accuser, which is the reverse of the norm in the American judicial system. All of these laws require the accuser to prove the truth of his or her statements, rather than requiring the corporations to prove the statements are false.

These were the laws used to bring a $10 million class action lawsuit against Oprah Winfrey when she said on national television that she was done eating hamburgers because of the possibility of getting "mad cow" disease. Oprah got in trouble with Texas beef producers, because she had the nerve to review former Montana cattle rancher Howard

Lyman's book, *Mad Cowboy: Plain Truth from the Cattle Rancher Who Won't Eat Meat,* on her nationally syndicated TV show.

Oprah Winfrey defeated the Texas cattlemen in court, but her legal fees were estimated at more than $1 million. This is another one of our corrupt "only in America" outcomes. You win your case against America's big corporate interests—but you lose a lot of your time and $1 million. I should point out here the average cost to each American is estimated to be $885 as your personal, out of pocket, annual subsidy to America's trial lawyers.

If I may digress for a moment, there are two legal reforms in America that are long overdue. The first is we need to go back to the English and Canadian system and not permit the gamesmanship contest of allowing lawyers to cherry pick juries that will try their case. This is a simple and easy reform to our legal system—you seat the first twelve qualified jurors and dismiss those with a close, personal connection to the case. How hard is that? Billions of dollars would be saved each year and millions of hours of time. The legal systems in Canada and England have proved there is little difference in the outcomes. The second simple change is adopting the time honored tradition of having the loser pay the court costs. Why shouldn't Oprah Winfrey be reimbursed for her legal fees by the Texas cattlemen who tried to shut her up for speaking her mind? Our legal system is so defective in America that even billionaires like Oprah get pushed around.

Corruption in the Food Industry

The food industry in America is currently America's biggest business. It's a trillion dollar annual business accounting for over 13% of the gross national product. About 17% of the labor force in America is involved in food production, manufacturing or distribution.

Some of the biggest budgets of the food giants are for advertising. The Pepsi Cola Corporation spends more than $1 billion each year advertising to sell you more foods loaded with high fructose corn syrup and hydrogenated oils. It's a fact that most advertising money goes to promote the most heavily processed foods. Because there's so much money at stake selling you junk food, it's hard getting independent opinions, even from magazines , such as *Journal of Nutrition Education, Journal of Nutrition,* and *American Journal of Clinical Nutrition.*

Independent opinions get compromised quickly when a publication's corporate sponsors include The Sugar Association, Gerber Foods, Coca-Cola, Proctor and Gamble and the Nestle/Carnation Corporation. Why would a company making food products as defective of those of the Coca-Cola Corporation give money to a nutritional journal, other than to influence the opinions of the journal editors?

It's hard finding a better example of how our nutritional authorities are corrupted by corporate payola than the story of the late Dr. Frederick Stare. In the 1950s, Dr. Stare left his Midwestern roots behind to become head of the nutrition department at Harvard University. He made this transition after a long career studying how nutritional deficiencies were caused by white flour, and a major factor in heart disease was consumption of vegetable oils. However, his beliefs underwent a sea change when he became the head of the nutrition department at Harvard. Soon, Harvard started receiving large grants from America's biggest business, the processed food industry, and Dr. Stare's newspaper columns began reassuring the public that sugar, white bread, and highly processed foods were just dandy for your health. He even advocated drinking one cup of corn oil daily to prevent heart disease! Dr. Stare proclaimed Coca-Cola was harmless and a few teaspoons of sugar in your coffee wouldn't hurt you, but would give you quick energy.

The Chemical Reality

There are enormous problems with agri-business in America, but you, the consumer, are the last to know. One of the perennial problems of American food production is the lack of government regulations of dangerous, toxic chemicals. Each year, over one billion pounds of pesticides are sprayed on food crops in America. According to the EPA, over 90% of fungicides, 60% of pesticides, and 30% of insecticides are known to be carcinogenic. Pesticide residues can be detected in over 50% of all foods in the U.S.

THE FACTS OF LIFE AND DEATH IN AMERICA
There are over 80,000 chemicals produced in North America.
Over 3,000 chemicals are added to our food supply.
Over 10,000 chemical solvents, emulsifiers, and preservatives are used in food production.
Over 1,000 new chemicals are introduced each year.

The bad news is that less than 3% of the 80,000 chemicals in use have ever been tested for safety. I thought of doing an A-Z list of them, but decided I'd give you just two on the A list that are some of the most dangerous and widely used chemical substances in our food chain.

✓ *Atrazine* is an extremely powerful herbicide whose use is ubiquitous in the growing of corn in America. Traces of this chemical can be found in streams and in well water and processed foods. It's often found in concentrations greater than 0.1 part per billion. Atrazine has recently been banned by the European Union because it's a suspected carcinogen and an endocrine disrupter linked to low sperm counts in farmers. A recent researcher at the University of Berkeley working for Syngenta, atrazine's manufacturer, found that concentrations of atrazine as low as 0.1 per billion will chemically emasculate a frog and cause its gonads to produce eggs. Atrazine turns male frogs into hermaphrodites. Perhaps the low sperm count in farmers exposed to Atrazine is nature's way of preventing birth defects in babies.

✓ **Acrylamides** are a group of chemicals used industrially in manufacturing some plastics. They're also formed when starches are heated. Three highly processed foods containing high levels of acrylamides are donuts, French fries, and potato chips. The maximum limit of acrylamides allowed by the EPA in your drinking water is 0.12 micrograms per serving. A six ounce serving of French fries at your favorite fast food joint contains 50 to 70 micrograms of acrylamides. That's over 400 to 600 times the EPA limits. I don't want you to think I'm telling you here that potatoes are a bad food—because they're not. Potatoes contain less than 1% fat, but when they're eaten as French fries cooked at a fast food joint with hydrogenated soybean oil, the fat content in your serving of potatoes can be increased as much as 200 times.

I won't go any further than the start of the A-list of chemicals in explaining why cancer is epidemic in America. Eliminating toxic chemicals in your food supply is one of the first baby steps you can take on the path to good health. Another is to realize that it takes the annual crop production of over two and a half acres of farmland to feed one American on a diet high in beef, Pringles, Sugar Smacks, Big Macs, Cheese Whiz and French fries. Obviously, one of the best things you can do to improve your own health and make a better environment is cut back drastically on your consumption of industrial beef.

The Impact of Industrial Beef

Probably the worst use of resources in America is the incredible damage done by industrial beef production. The introduction of cattle breeds native to moist climates of northern Europe to Western range lands has had disastrous effects upon these naturally dry Western lands. The open range lands of the American West are Ground Zero for the most devastating effects of beef production. The West has truly been wasted to produce only a tiny amount of American beef.

Probably the worst example of this effect is the damage caused by more than 1,000 ranchers who graze cattle on dry public lands in Arizona. They have more control over using the land than the other 5 million people in Arizona. It's hard to believe, but in California over 100 ranchers still have active cattle leases in the bone-dry Mojave Desert. The U. S. Treasury spends over $1 billion annually in subsidies to Western cattle producers, producing less than 3% of America's beef.

It's time to phase out grazing on public lands in the American west and start using them for higher and better uses, like raising wildlife or using these lands for recreation. As writer Lynn Jacobs said in her book, *Waste of the West: Public Lands Ranching*, "Ranching has wasted and is wasting the United States more than any other human endeavor." Government supported "welfare ranching" has reduced the biological productivity of the American West by over 90%, since grazing started 150 years ago. The average range-fed steer consumes six tons of vegetation annually before going to slaughter. Raising beef on Western grazing lands has proven to be a stupid use of most of the West's dry and fragile land. In Iowa, a cow only needs to graze one acre to survive, a cow in Alabama needs three acres, and on Western range lands, each cow needs at least 185 acres to graze at the public's expense.

At least half of U.S. rangeland in the mountainous western states is now considered "severely degraded." In the western states such as Idaho, Colorado, Arizona and New Mexico, most of the riparian zones by western streams have been degraded beyond nature's capacity to repair them. Cattle have largely replaced buffalo, deer, elk, moose, bighorn sheep and other large herbivores that used to live in Western North America in much greater numbers. Their numbers have now been reduced by cattle and sheep ranching to less than 3% of their original populations.

Surprisingly enough, you would think that the National Wildlife Refuges would be places where wildlife would be protected. Actually, of the 109 Wildlife Refuges in Wyoming, Montana, Colorado, Utah, Kansas, Nebraska and the Dakotas, 103 of them allow cattle grazing. More than half of the West's topsoil has been lost since grazing started about 150 years ago.

Livestock has also spread many diseases into the wildlife population such as anthrax, brucellosis, pinkeye, scabies, encephalitis, and leptospirosis. Most of the buffalo and elk in the state of Wyoming are infected with brucellosis, contracted from strains introduced by cattle. To control brucellosis, some in the ranching community feel all elk and buffalo in Wyoming should be killed and replaced with strains of wild animals that are certified brucellosis free!

The energy and water inputs into raising Western cattle on dry land defy common sense. This is a product that wouldn't be produced if it wasn't being generously (and foolishly) subsidized by the U.S. taxpayer. Currently, it takes about 16 pounds of grain to make one pound of beef, and 80% of American grain production goes to feed animals. How many more people could we feed if we all ate a little further down the food chain?

Water is the lifeblood of the American West and water is being used and abused by ranching interests to produce surplus beef at an incredible environmental cost. Over 70% of the water resources of the 11 Western states are used for raising livestock. In Montana, over 97% of water production goes to raise livestock. In Arizona and the Northwest states, over 50% of water use is committed to raising livestock. The amount of water needed to produce ten pounds of steak equals the annual water consumption of the average household. Overall, the American taxpayer has subsidized this destruction of the American West to benefit a handful of livestock producers. Federal money has paid for over half of all irrigation projects in the Western states.

Without the technology of drilling deep water wells and using petroleum products on a huge scale, the American West would never have developed such widespread production of the grain being grown to feed cattle. We in America have lived a lifestyle subsidized by the blessings bestowed upon us by the Ogallala Aquifer, the largest underground lake ever discovered on planet Earth. This gigantic underground lake reaching from Nebraska to Texas was created by millions of years of rainwater seeping down into the earth to form an immense underground reservoir.

The bad news is that this aquifer is being depleted, like our once abundant and cheap supplies of petroleum, at a reckless pace, and will be mostly exhausted within the next 50 years. Already, around the margins of the Ogallala Aquifer in Texas, Missouri, Colorado and Nebraska, the cost of deeper and deeper wells is putting grain farmers out of business. Fields that were green and lush are now being taken out of production and are going back to being a part of the dusty, Western landscape.

American Agri-Business and Oil

Not just the American West, but all large scale agriculture is critically dependent upon access to cheap and abundant petroleum and natural gas resources that no longer exist. America's oil resources peaked out in 1971 and have been in sharp decline ever since. Despite that hard fact, we're still the world's most reckless and profligate consumers of oil, with average consumption of petroleum products of over three gallons per person in America each day of the year. On a world scale, the average Italian burns about 1.4 gallons of oil daily, South Africans and Brazilians burn about .5 gallons and the average person in China consumes .15 gallons daily, according to a report by the *World News Network*.

Every day as an American, you're enjoying the benefits of the bounty of cheap petroleum that has fueled the rise in unsustainable lifestyles such as the production of cheap beef, pork, chicken and eggs. At least 20% of America's arable lands are currently planted in corn, which requires extremely high amounts of petroleum-based fertilizers and pesticides. It takes as much as a half gallon of oil to grow each bushel of corn. There are real environmental and social costs to the seemingly endless cornucopia of cheap food that American Agri-Business has created. Any steps you take towards buying food that's locally produced and grown is good for your health and good for the planet, too.

A great deal of the world's oil production is currently coming from a small number of some of the largest oil fields ever discovered in Saudi Arabia, Kuwait, and Mexico. Some industry experts feel peak oil has been reached in these fields. Like all other large deposits ever discovered, such as Prudhoe Bay in Alaska and the North Sea oil fields, once peak production is obtained, fast declines in production are inevitable. The year 1988 was the last year in which the world discovered as much oil as was consumed. Globally, with the industrialization of China and India occurring simultaneously, the world is consuming five to six times as much new oil each year as is being discovered.

You might have heard the news of immense oil deposits being discovered in the Gulf of Mexico in 2006. That's good news for our oil driven economy and lifestyle, but the bad news is just how far we have to go to get that oil. The large scale discoveries in the Gulf of Mexico were in waters 8,000 to 10,000 deep, and the drill strings discovering and bringing up these oil deposits went down another four or five miles into the earth's crust, once the sea floor was pierced. I mention this to underscore the lengths and depths we're going to in squeezing the last drops from the earth. There's just no easy or cheap oil left.

There is nothing sustainable about America's insatiable thirst for this inky, condensed, black juice of the ancient swamps where dinosaurs once roamed. Within our lifetime, the American lifestyle and agricultural practices are both reaching the limits of exploitation.

Cheap and Toxic Manufactured Food

Food is big business, but the largest profits in American food production aren't made from raising food. The biggest profit margins come but from getting you, the consumer, to purchase food products manufactured from cheap commodities.

One of the worst offenders in the American diet is white flour. According to an FDA analysis of nutrients, refined white flour has 77% less fiber, 21% less protein and 54% less calcium than whole grain flours. Along with the missing nutrients, almost all processed foods are drastically lacking in fiber. Whole grain pasta has three times as much fiber as pasta made from refined flour, and brown rice has four times as much fiber as white rice.

Last year, over half a million people in the U.S. were hospitalized for *diverticulitis*, which is an intestinal disease caused primarily by not eating enough fiber. This is an All-American disease, almost completely unknown elsewhere in the world, that is caused by excess consumption of processed foods. In addition to protecting you from diverticulitis, one of the bonuses of eating soluble fiber found in beans, barley, oats, whole wheat, vegetables and fruits, is that a high fiber diet also suppresses your appetite. Fiber gives you a feeling of fullness and helps you avoid overeating.

American food processors can make almost anything from the Holy Trinity of hydrogenated soybean oil, white sugar, and white flour. Look closely at the ingredients in many of today's snack and convenience foods and you'll realize these three ingredients are the basic feed stock for many products. Different flavors—same ingredients.

I've always wondered if certain products actually had highly addictive ingredients that food manufacturers don't want you to know about. What food additive is in Chicken-In-A Biscuit crackers, BBQ potato chips, Pringles, and Wheat-Thins that makes you unable to eat just one of them? I've always suspected they put something more powerful than salt and sugar in them. Is there an ingredient X in these highly addictive foods?

When I grew up in the 1950s, my favorite food was a type of candy called Lik-M-Ade. It was a brightly colored, sugar and chemical powder that you poured into your hand and licked up with your tongue. A large percentage of my cavities probably started with my using this doozy of a candy product.

Cereal Story

My favorite breakfast cereal back in the '50s was Sugar Smacks. Occasionally I'd eat Corn Pops, but my mainstay was Sugar Smacks, a product known to be 56% sugar. Just the thing to sit down with and watch Howdy Doody, Sky King, Sea Hunt, and Davey Crockett on that old time black and white TV. I realize I'm dating myself here, but I was a mere 13 years old when the Beatles first strummed their guitars, beat their drums, and sang their magic songs on the Ed Sullivan Show. If you're anywhere near my age, keep reading! You might need this health information to make sure you're still on the right side of the green grass!

Researching this book, I discovered that not only are all puffed cereal products unhealthy—they're actually toxic to your health. The first health food advocate to publicize this was Paul Stitt who wrote *Fighting the Food Giants* in the early 1980s. Before Stitt quit the corporate world and started one of the first all-natural bakeries in Wisconsin over 30 years ago, he worked for some of America's biggest corporations as a biochemist involved in manufacturing foods. At his last job at Quaker Oats, Stitt came across a flyer in Quaker's library that had been published in 1942. It was a report of a study in which four sets of rats had been given special diets (see Box: RATS FED ON PUFFED GRAINS).

RATS FED ON PUFFED GRAINS	
RATS WERE FED:	LIFE SPAN:
Water, vitamins, whole wheat kernels	They lived for over one year.
Water and vitamins	They lived eight weeks.
White Sugar and Water	They lived four weeks.
Puffed Wheat, Water and vitamins	They only lived two weeks!

What this study suggested was that the rats weren't dying of malnutrition, but rather, there was something extremely toxic about grains that have been puffed by a high heat process and made into a food. As a biochemist, Paul Stitt stated proteins are similar to toxins in molecular structure, and perhaps the process of puffing wheat grains with 1,500 pounds per square inch of pressure might have turned a nutritious grain into a toxic substance.

And Quaker Oats has known about this since the early 1940s! Paul Stitt got nowhere confronting management about his discovery, and he eventually left Quaker to start his own whole grain bakery in Wisconsin. You won't catch me eating any of Quaker's hugely successful puffed rice products that you can buy down at your local grocery store.

Recently some grains of red wheat were found in an Egyptian tomb belonging to the king Tutankhamen, and researchers were still able to sprout them, even though they were 3,000 years old. Obviously, if you want to be a healthy human being you have to eat real, *live* foods, not *ersatz* American manufactured foods. Most of the people in the world are much healthier than Americans, and they live primarily on green leafy vegetables, grains, beans, peas, lentils, lots of fruit and vegetables and small amounts of meat and fish.

When to it comes to bad health, the really bad food products are the ubiquitous high fructose corn syrup, hydrogenated oils, refined white flours and sugar that are found everywhere in American foods. If you want to be a healthy human being, don't eat them. Products that contain them are not foods—no matter how much food manufacturers would like you to believe they are.

Trans Fats and Fake Fats

The scientific evidence is beginning to accumulate, showing just how dangerous hydrogenated trans fats in cheap products like Crisco are for your health. Trans fats and hydrogenated oils interfere with cell membrane functions, interfere with the enzyme systems your body needs to eliminate carcinogens and toxins, inhibit insulin receptors, and decrease hormone production. They are strongly linked to cancer, diabetes and infertility. Sadly, trans fats in the diets of pregnant women contribute to low birth weight babies and can inhibit visual and neurological functions. They also lower fat content in mother's milk and depress learning ability.

As I mentioned in Chapter Two, you need to eat healthy saturated fats from natural sources such as olive oil, butter, coconut oil, beef tallow and lard. They're much better for you than polyunsaturated vegetable oils, hydrogenated soybean oil and trans-fats. Today, the European countries with the highest levels of consumption of saturated fats—Switzerland, the Netherlands, France, Belgium, Finland and Austria—have the lowest levels of heart disease. The countries with the lowest levels of saturated fat consumption—Ukraine, Croatia, Macedonia, Tajikistan and Georgia—have the highest rates of heart disease.

The reason, of course, why most manufactured foods contain hydrogenated oils and trans-fats is that they give products like Crisco a shelf life from here to eternity. And of course, America's food manufacturers are always working overtime developing new products to help you eat as much as you like, yet not consume very much fat. One of their latest trick products was the approval of Olestra, a newly engineered "miracle fat" in 1998. This is a Proctor and Gamble product that is actually a *polyester sucrose*, which is a mixture of cottonseed and soybean oils around a core of sugar. (Hmmm—is this a food—or a formula for polyester pants?)

The beauty of Olestra (it helps to be a shareholder of Proctor and Gamble to see *beauty* here!) is that your body wants nothing to do with this chemical. It goes it one end, you get the pleasant "mouthfeel," and it comes out the other end.

Sounds beautiful, doesn't it? You get to eat fat and not get fat. One of the minor problems with Olestra is it takes fat soluble vitamins and beta carotenes along with it when it leaves. The manufacturers of food containing Olestra have to warn you to supplement your diet with vitamins if you eat foods containing Olestra. Thanks for the "help" with our diet, Proctor and Gamble!

CHAPTER ELEVEN

Food That's Good For You To Eat

I'm glad you've come this far along the path and stuck with me through the doom and gloom tale of the myriad interlocking scams in America in agri-business, Big Pharma, and Big Medicine. I hope the many stories in this book have already encouraged you to seek out healthy foods and eat as naturally as you can, Now, in this chapter, I'm going to tell you what foods will nourish you and help you live a long and healthy life.

Basic Advice for Healthy Eating

Bottom line, grow your own food whenever you can and always try to buy locally produced, organic food. Eating foods that are fresh, local, and in season is critical to your good health. Support your local farmers every chance you get. I can't emphasize enough the dual nature of our food situation here in America: Natural foods that should be good for you are not, because they have been damaged by profit-motivated growing, manufacturing, and processing practices. Stay away from foods that are produced with your best interest low on the list!

In figuring out what foods make us healthy, we need to remember there are a lot of different people all over the world living healthy lives while eating extremely different diets than our American diet. Here and abroad, people of different cultures have developed an enormous variety of cuisines from what nature has offered them. When it comes to food, there are few limits to human ingenuity. Who am I to tell people in other cultures that their unique foods aren't good for them? I'm not about to tell the Mexicans that their chocolate mole sauce or their smoky, chipotle chile sauces on their roasted chicken isn't good for them. Or should I tell the Vietnamese that their pungent, salty fish sauces aren't good to eat in their steaming hot bowls of Pho? In many cases, their cuisines are healthier by far than ours! I urge you to enjoy some of the beneficial effects of globalization and enjoy the special foods of many cultures. Welcome to the positive, synergistic events unfolding in America's mighty, multi-cultural future!

But I do stay away from convenience foods. I used to occasionally eat at fast food restaurants, as many of my fellow Americans do every day, but after discovering what I did in writing this book, you won't find me standing in line at Mickey D's any more. What I've learned is this: If you see the Golden Arches too often, it won't be long before you see the Pearly Gates.

Probably the best advice I can give you is to follow in the footsteps of healthy primitives and eat a lot of fruits and vegetables, eat some meats and fish raw, and be sure to partake of soups and broths made from beef, chicken, or fish bones. Unlike the absurdity of high protein diets or low carbohydrate diets, the Santa Barbara Diet is *high in carbohydrates and rich in fiber*, with a variable amount of protein that you determine your body needs.

Bear in mind however, that most Americans eat from two to four times more protein than they need. Experiment with your diet and find out how much protein you should eat. I think a diet very high in protein is fine—but only if you're going to physically exert yourself strenuously for five or six hours every day. Looking around at my fellow Americans, I don't see too many of us in that category. How much effort did it take to check your messages on your Blackberry, turn on your computer, or turn on your car's ignition switch? It's true that affluence can kill you.....

Healthiest Food Picks

The rest of this chapter is about the best possible foods to eat for nutrition and for good health. What follows is my recommendations for foods from Asian cuisines and from more traditional American cuisines (both Native and 21st century), as well as those from Africa, the Middle East, and Europe.

My highest recommendation goes to the cuisines of Vietnam and Thailand for being among the world's healthiest cuisines. These two countries, along with the Philippine Islands, have the world's lowest rates of cancer and heart disease. It's widely believed by many that the large amount of coconut oil consumed is a major factor in their good health.

I hope by now I've convinced you that high quality saturated fats should be an important part of your diet. Heart disease was virtually unknown in America when saturated fats made up the majority of the fats consumed. Coconut oil, olive oil and butter are the very best oils for your health. Don't eat *any* polyunsaturated vegetable oils, such as soybean oil, safflower oil, sunflower oil, corn oil, cottonseed oil and canola oil. Polyunsaturated oil is a product promoted by America's food manufacturing industry when the supply of coconut oil dried up at the start of World War II. Their widespread use has been a major factor in America's heart disease epidemic that peaked in 1968.

I'm going to start out this saga of what's good for you by explaining some of the key elements in the cuisine of Vietnam and Thailand, two countries that have the world's healthiest diets.

COCONUT OIL

The beauty of coconut oil, especially for those trying to lose weight, is that it is a medium chain fatty acid and works differently in your body than other oils do. Unlike soybean oil, it has no negative effects on your thyroid gland and actually speeds up your metabolism to help you lose weight.

Some coconut oils in our modern world have been hydrogenated, and you should avoid them like the plague. Because coconut oil is such a highly saturated fat, it's the least vulnerable of all the cooking oils to oxidation and free radical formation, and it's the safest to use in cooking. Virgin, unprocessed coconut oil will melt at 76 degrees (25C), and that's how you can tell if it's been hydrogenated. Hydrogenated coconut stays liquid up to 95 degrees. Do not use hydrogenated coconut oils. They're just as bad for you as hydrogenated soybean oils.

Over 80% of all vegetable oils in the United States are dangerous hydrogenated or partially hydrogenated oils. One of American food processors' favorite tricks is to sell you soybean oil by giving it a marketing name, like Wesson Oil. Another trick is to blend soybean oil with cheaper oils, like those made from cottonseed. Do your health a favor and go around your house, identify such oils and throw them in the trash can. Replace them with coconut oil, and eat at all you want of this natural health food.

The early explorers of the South Pacific were amazed at the beauty, good health and physical vitality of the native people, most of whom had coconut oil as the mainstay of their diet. In some primitive cultures, coconut oil has comprised as much as 60% of the total intake of calories, and these are some of the healthiest people you could find anywhere. Heart disease and cancer were completely unknown in traditional Polynesian culture.

Over the few years I've been writing this book, I've seen how coconut oil is starting to catch on. Once you start using it, you'll quickly reject the dietary dogma that coconut oil and saturated fats are bad for you. Coconut oil is on the FDA's list of GRAS (Generally Regarded As Safe) substances and is considered a safe, natural food. It is a key component of many hospital formulas to feed critically ill patients, and is a major part of baby formulas, because it provides many of the same nutrients as human breast milk.

Many of the health benefits of coconut oil come from the high ratio of lauric acid (as much as 48%) in its unique composition of medium chain fatty acids. Lauric acid has been proven to have powerful antibacterial, antifungal, anti-parasitic, and antiviral properties. The lauric acid in coconut oil is a medium chain fatty acid designed by nature to give you quick energy, just like the large amounts of lauric acid in human breast milk.

Many of those afflicted with Crohn's disease have found coconut oil to have powerful effects in naturally healing this autoimmune disease. Also, because of the beneficial effects for men of the fatty acids in saw palmetto berries used for prostate problems, it's quite likely that the medium chain fatty acids in coconut oil have similar properties. In Thailand, where they have the highest per capita consumption of coconuts, they also have the lowest cancer rates of 50 countries surveyed in a recent study. When it comes to your health, coconut oil is the best oil in the world.

SPROUTS

In Asian cuisines from China to Vietnam to Malaysia, you'll find sprouts made from seeds and beans are commonly used in many different types of dishes from stir fry to spring rolls. This is because sprouts are full of vital enzymes, amino acids, vitamins and minerals. Commonly used mung bean sprouts are a good source of protein, high in vitamin C, and rich in iron and potassium. Try using young mung bean sprouts mixed with steamed rice and sauces for a Thai style nutritional boost.

Eating a certain amount of your diet as living food is one of the best things you can do for good health. Sprouting seeds increases enzyme activity as much as six times. The American diet is lacking in enzymes. and eating raw foods helps your blood become more alkaline versus the toxic acidity of a high protein diet. Sprouting seeds also increases vitamin B and C content, and the carotene (vitamin A) content can increase as much as eight times. Sprouted grains of all types are good for you.

LEMONS, LIMES, AND GRAPEFRUITS

Lemons are native to South East Asia and were only introduced to the Mediterranean areas around 1000 AD. All of these fruits are used widely in Asian cuisines and are extremely good for you. Botanically, these fruits are classified as acid fruits, but when they're digested in your stomach, they have an alkaline effect upon your system. The American diet is 80% acidic and less than 20% alkaline, which is the opposite of what it should be. See Chapter Eight for the relative alkalinity or acidity of various foods, and how this impacts your health.

Lemon and lime juices have anti-microbial properties, and their high acidity make them perfect for marinating raw fish. All three of these fruits have very low sugar levels. Lemons and limes have 3% and grapefruit has 5% sugar. Add these fruit juices to water for a nourishing healthy drink, as they are all powerful anti-oxidants.

BANANAS

Bananas are a central part of all Asian cuisines, and many different types are eaten. There are good reasons for their wide consumption because they have many beneficial health effects. Bananas are high in fiber and the natural sugars of fructose and glucose. Bananas also contain *tryptophan,* which is a type of protein your body converts into the brain chemical *serotonin.* You want to have high levels of serotonin, because it is a natural mood elevator and counters depression. Also, the vitamin B6 in bananas helps regulate your glucose levels.

Because bananas are so high in potassium and low in sodium, it is believed they help reduce your blood pressure, and as part of a daily routine, can actually reduce your risk of stroke. Compared to apples, they have four times the protein, twice the carbohydrates, three times the phosphorus, five times the vitamin A and iron and up to twice the levels of other vitamins and trace minerals.

EGGS

Chickens were first domesticated thousands of years ago in South East Asia, and the cuisines of Vietnam, Thailand, China, and Malaysia use eggs extensively. Eggs from free range chickens are among the healthiest, most complete and economical protein source available. Never let the dietary nonsense about eggs being high in cholesterol keep you from eating eggs from healthy free range chickens raised on high quality feed. Every 24 hours, your body produces about 3,000 milligrams of cholesterol (about the amount in 10 eggs) no matter what you eat. This occurs regardless of how much dietary cholesterol you ingest. Make sure you eat eggs from free range chickens—their eggs are much more nutritious than those from industrial chickens.

FISH SAUCE AND SESAME SEEDS

Fish sauce is an important ingredient in both Vietnamese and Thai cuisine that has synergistic effects in your diet to help you absorb vitamins and minerals more efficiently. Traditional fish sauces give complex, rich, salty flavors to food, and like their nutritional components, they add up to more than the sum of the parts. A completely natural product, fish sauce is made by soaking small fish in wooden barrels with salt and water, and then letting them ferment for months. Rich in B vitamins and with small amounts of protein, fish sauces are a key part of the nutritional synergies in Thai and Vietnamese food.

Sesame seeds are used in many types of Asian cuisines for very good reasons. They have a unique protein composition that contains large amounts of *methionine* and *tryptophan*, both amino acids that are missing from almost all other vegetable protein sources. These amino acids are important for liver and kidney functions and the utilization of B vitamins. Sesame seeds also have high amounts of calcium, phosphorus, vitamin B, iron, and potassium. Eat them ground and sprinkled on your rice and vegetable dishes, or as *tahini*, a sesame butter or paste that can be made into a sauce or spread.

NUTS

Raw, unsalted nuts give your body high quality oils, trace minerals, and vitamins. The widespread use of chopped peanuts in Thai and Vietnamese foods came about because of peanut's richness in available nutrients. Nuts are among the most nutrient dense of all foods. They are rich sources of natural oil, some containing 60% to 80% of their calories as fat. Nuts are also an excellent natural source of *boron*, an important trace mineral needed for good bone health. It's believed that boron helps stimulate hormones that play an important role in bone growth. Recent studies giving post-menopausal women boron supplements reduced their calcium and magnesium losses, and increased their estrogen levels. Peanuts, almonds, and hazelnuts have high levels of boron. Among fruits, good sources of boron are apples, pears and tomatoes.

Studies have shown that eating an ounce of nuts twice a week reduces the rate of coronary heart disease by 30%. My guess is these benefits occur because of the abundant trace minerals in nuts that are so lacking in the American diet. It's also possible the fatty acids and calcium in nuts help prevent disease.

HERE IS A LIST OF THE NUTRITIONAL CONTENTS IN THE MOST COMMON NUTS:
Sunflower seeds are 27% protein with lots of calcium, iron, phosphorus, potassium, and magnesium. They are also good sources of B vitamins and carotenoids.
Pumpkin seeds are high in zinc, iron, and Omega 3 and Omega 6 oils.

Pecans come from a tree with very deep roots which can grow to 150 feet and produce up to 200 pounds of nuts each year. They are high in calcium, iron, phosphorus, potassium, magnesium, and selenium. Like blueberries, they're exceptionally rich in manganese.

Walnuts are high in iron, magnesium, zinc, phosphorus, and potassium. Ounce for ounce, walnuts contain equal amounts of calories as butter and bacon. They're 60% fat and high in Omega 3 oils. But these oils go rancid very quickly, so ideally, you should only eat walnuts you have shelled yourself. Shelled walnut meats should always be refrigerated or stored in a freezer. Walnut oil is delicious and highly nutritious; however, it should never be heated.

Cashews are the nut of a pear size fruit native to Brazil. Grown extensively in India too, they're rich in protein, magnesium, and phosphorus and potassium. They're low in fat compared to most nuts.

Brazil nuts contain selenium, an important antioxidant mineral, that's deficient in North American soils. You can get the recommended amount of 200 micrograms by eating two Brazil nuts daily. Don't eat too many, though— excess selenium isn't good for you.

Macadamia nuts are Queensland's gift to the world. They're rich in minerals, such as iron, copper, magnesium, zinc, phosphorus and potassium. They're also high in B vitamins and have a unique fatty acids profile. My favorite way to eat macadamia nuts is use them finely ground and mixed with Panko crumbs—a Japanese style bread crumb typically used on pork, chicken or fish—on a tasty fish, like onaga, the deep-water Hawaiian red snapper. Want to try it? I recommend you go to Mama's Fish House near Paia on the island of Maui to experience the celestial mingling of flavors from Queensland and Maui.

For the rest of this chapter, I'm detouring away from the Asian slant on health foods and going on to the traditional ways of health from Native American, European, Middle Eastern, African and 21st century food knowledge to explain the healthiest foods you can eat.

BUFFALO, WILD GAME, AND ORGANIC BEEF

I think the world's finest meat is buffalo tenderloin cooked medium rare and topped with a Swedish style lingonberry sauce. A close second

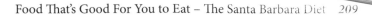

would be buffalo short ribs with a good homemade barbecue sauce. Last year, I again bought half a buffalo from a ranch near Ucross, Wyoming. It was a two year old heifer that had primarily been raised on grass. She was finished off with corn and alfalfa hay, and I paid $4 per pound.

Organic, grass fed buffalo and prime beef are the meats of both the past and the future. Do your part to support buffalo ranchers whenever you can. Buffalo is the natural beef, a perfectly evolved and adapted animal for the high Western grasslands of North America.

There are many good reasons to add buffalo meat to your diet. Buffalo is high in protein, low in cholesterol, and extremely high in Omega 3 oils. Eating buffalo meat can help you balance out one of the unhealthiest parts of the American diet—the enormous imbalance of Omega 6 to Omega 3 oils. Eating meat from industrial beef with an unnaturally skewed ratio of Omega 6 to Omega 3 oils is an unhealthy component of the American diet. (However, the primary reason for the imbalance is probably the dangerous and unhealthy use of vegetable oils such as soy, corn, safflower, and canola oils.) Recent studies from North Dakota State University showed that grass-fed buffalo has an Omega 6 to Omega 3 oil ratio of 4:1. After 200 days in a feed lot, grain-fed cattle had an Omega 6 to Omega 3 oil ratio of 20:1. Buffalo meat has as much as 35% more protein than beef and twice the beta-carotene and iron.

Buffalo are one of the few land animals that do not get cancer. Some researchers speculate this may be because their meat is high in *conjugated linolenic acid* (CLA) which is found in high levels in the butterfat of dairy cows. In lab testing at the University of Wisconsin at Madison, researchers found CLA seems to offer protection against breast cancer, prevent the deposition of fat, and increase milk production. CLA is only found in high levels in cows that graze on green grass.

Buffalo also have a lot of unique traits that make them much better for the Western landscape than beef cattle. Unlike cows, they don't congregate at water holes, they drop their calves with no assistance, and they don't despoil pastures because they keep moving. Also, they're hardy enough to survive the most extreme winters on the Northern Plains without protection or care. Pull a nickel out of your pocket and take a look—the American Bison—God's Cow!

All wild game is extremely high in Omega 6 oils and low in fat. Almost any kind of wild game you can eat is nutritionally superior to farm raised animals. It's hard to improve upon nature. If beef is raised properly upon good pasture and not laced with antibiotics, steroids, or growth hormones—it's an excellent food. But how much of American's beef production fits that criteria. My guess is less than 1%!

BEANS

Almost all types of beans— peas, beans, and lentils—are among the best foods you can eat. Beans are high in zinc, calcium, magnesium, folic acid, B vitamins, fiber, protein, and complex carbohydrates. The nutritional powerhouse of the bean family is the tiny lentil. Lentils are high in phosphorus, calcium, magnesium, zinc, iron, B vitamin complex, and molybdenum. Eating lentils, very fresh vegetables, lots of butter, and organ meats are key elements in French cuisine and a major factor in French people's low levels of heart disease. Use red lentils for soups and try the tiny green lentils the French love so much. You would have to eat 7½ pounds of potatoes, 11 pounds of beets or 9½ pounds of carrots to get the amount of phosphorus in one pound of lentils.

SWEET POTATOES

Sweet potatoes are one of the only foods you could live on without eating anything else. They are the most nutritious of all vegetables and they're full of iron, calcium, magnesium, potassium, B6, vitamin C, fiber and beta-carotene. The carotene content of sweet potatoes actually increases when they're stored during the winter. Our bodies can only convert beta-carotene into much needed vitamin A in the presence of bile salts. That's why it's important to eat cream, butter, egg yolks or coconut oil with sweet potatoes to help stimulate your secretions of bile. And you thought this book was going to give you some sort of severe dietary regimen? Eat your coconut cream and your maple syrup with your sweet potatoes. It's good for you….

BEETS

Beets are nutritional powerhouses. They contain large amounts of iron, copper, calcium, phosphorus, potassium, carotene, B complex vitamins and vitamin C. Both beets and their green tops contain special substances that stimulate your liver and the flow of bile juices. Beets are sometimes used in manufacturing natural vitamins. They have long been valued as a springtime tonic for the blood.

PRUNES

Prunes are high in iron and they have the highest amounts of antioxidant phytochemicals of any fruit. They're high in vitamin A and potassium too. High quality dried plums are one of the most power packed foods you can eat. The Japanese revere many types of plums for very good reasons.

AVOCADOS

Avocados are extremely high in folic acid, magnesium, vitamin A, B vitamins, iron, and trace minerals. They contain some of the healthiest plant oils you can eat. A recent study done at Ohio State University showed that you need fat with vegetables to help you absorb vitamins. This research showed that men and women eating salsa with added avocado absorbed 4.4 time as much lycopenes and 2.6 times as much beta carotene as eating salsa without avocado. This effect was even more pronounced when avocado was added to a salad containing shredded baby carrots, spinach, romaine lettuce and a 2% low fat dressing. In the study, when 11 people consumed this salad with avocado added, on average they absorbed seven times as much lutein and 18 times as much beta-carotene. Any type of healthy saturated fat, such as butter, olive oil, or coconut oil appears to have this effect. However, a German study with lab rats showed that eating hydrogenated oils with vegetables actually impeded absorption of vitamin E.

Of course, almost all industrial salad dressings sold in America contain hydrogenated soybean oils! As natural vitamin E has been shown to be very important for the good health of your heart, here's yet another defective American eating habit that can harm the health of those even trying to eat more vegetables! The message is clear: Eat healthy fats with your veggies to supercharge your nutrition. Make your own salad dressing with olive oil, lemon, lime, and natural sweeteners and herbs. If you're tempted to buy manufactured salad dressing for convenience, check the ingredients and only buy products that contain olive oil with no other oil added.

QUINOA, TEFF, AMARANTH, HEMP, AND CHIA

Quinoa (pronounced *keen-wa*) is an ancient grain that originated in the Andean region of South America where it has been cultivated for over 6,000 years. Quinoa can be grown up to 12,000 feet of elevation, and it's a hardy, prolific plant that was named *chisaya mama,* or "mother of all grains," by the Incas. Traditionally, the Inca emperor would sow the first seeds of the season using farming tools made of solid gold.

Quinoa has been designated as a super crop by the United Nations, because it has the highest protein content (12-18%) of any grain. Quinoa's protein is of an unusually high quality—it has a full complement of amino acids, very similar to the gold standard of amino acids, which is certified raw milk. Quinoa is a good source of dietary fiber, and is high in phosphorus, iron, and magnesium. Traditionally quinoa has been eaten in Andean cultures by nursing mothers, as it is reputed to increase the flow of breast milk. Quinoa is easy to cook, tastes good, and is an excellent substitute for couscous. In its natural state, the tiny seeds have a coating of bitter tasting *saponins* that need to be removed by soaking. In nature, these saponins prevent against the seeds being eaten by birds or insects. There are good recipes in the last chapter for quinoa, teff, and amaranth.

Teff is another ancient grain from the highlands of Ethiopia, where it's used to make a flat, tasty bread named *injera.* Teff is also cooked in porridge, eaten in stews, and used as a healthy additive to pancakes or waffles here in America. Use small amounts of teff flour to add nutrition to comfort foods like waffles. Teff is the world's smallest grain, but it has a tremendous nutritional profile with extremely high levels of calcium, phosphorus, iron, and other trace minerals.

Amaranth is another ancient grain that has been grown in many parts of the world. It was a favorite of both the Incas and the Aztecs who ate it toasted like popcorn and blended with honey for a healthy snack food. It has a complete complement of amino acids and is extremely high in calcium and manganese with high levels of iron, magnesium, phosphorus, and copper. In the Caribbean, amaranth leaves are used in a traditional soup called *callaloo*.

Hemp was first cultivated in China over 6,000 years ago—long before soybeans were grown. Hemp seed is now beginning to be sold in the U.S. in cereal and is crushed for nutritional oils. Hemp is high in digestible protein with a good balance of all eight essential amino acids. Hemp has three times as much vitamin E as flax, and twice the iron and magnesium.

Chia is another ancient food that was used by Native Americans for centuries. It was primarily used by the Aztecs and by Southwestern Indian tribes. It is extremely high in protein, contains all the amino acids, and has the highest levels of Omega 3 oils of any plant. Your body converts the Omega 3 oils in chia seeds into EPA and DHA. One ounce of chia seeds contains 2% B2 (riboflavin), 13% thiamin, and trace amounts of all B vitamins. Ounce for ounce, chia has three times more iron than spinach, five times more calcium than milk, and fifteen times more magnesium than broccoli. Chia is also super high in fiber and absorbs 30 times its weight in water. As a dieting aid, you put one tablespoon of chia seeds in eight ounces of water or orange juice, and let it sit for five minutes. Stir a few times, then drink it down. The high fiber helps clean your intestines and the chia helps you feel full for hours. It's a great, nutritional aid for dieters.

BREWER'S YEAST

Dried nutritional yeast, known as brewer's yeast, is extremely high in B complex vitamins and many minerals. It is also high in chromium, which all diabetics need. Seek out yeast processed at low temperatures and available at your local health food store in bins. It should be a light yellow color and dissolve quickly in liquid. Brewer's yeast is high in glutamic acid and it helps depress cravings for sugar and alcohol. Almost all animal and pet foods contain adequate amounts of brewer's yeast, the secret ingredient that gives Fido a shiny coat and thick fur.

WHEATGRASS

If you need to do some serious healing or cleansing, it's hard to find anything better for you than wheatgrass. This is a uniquely American health food, the use of which dates back to the early 1930s. Wheatgrass is one of the most powerful healing agents known. It contains more than 100 food elements, including every identified trace mineral and vitamin and every vitamin in the B vitamin complex. Wheatgrass is 25% protein and contains 17 amino acids. Wheatgrass neutralizes toxins and has a composition similar to human blood. It's a nutrient rich food that is among the best possible sources of chlorophyll.

The juicing of wheat, barley, and oat grasses was started by an out of work agricultural chemist from Kansas named Charles Schnabel. In the 1930s, Schnabel started experimenting with recipes to nurse ailing chickens back to good health. (In this digital age, do you know anyone with enough time on their hands to figure out how to nurse ailing chickens back to health?) Schnabel discovered miraculous results by feeding his chickens freshly cut young oat and wheat grasses. He realized he was on the right track one morning when he got 126 eggs from 106 hens.

The most powerful healing effects come when the juice is squeezed from wheatgrass just as it makes the first joint. The reason why cats or dogs chew on green grasses when they're sick or don't have an appetite is because grass contains very nutritious substances. For the same reason, in the springtime, when grizzly bears come out of their dens, they'll eat grass just like cows do.

I try and take a shot of wheatgrass every time I go to a farmer's market and can get it fresh. If you really need a good cleanse or have need of healing, consider growing and juicing wheatgrass yourself. It's easy and fun to do.

CHLORELLA AND SPIRULINA

Chlorella is a single cell algae that contains more chlorophyll per gram than any other substance. As a food supplement, it helps your liver detoxify and purify your blood. Chlorella helps balance your pH levels, stimulates production of red blood cells, and is especially good for removing heavy metals from your system. A recent study in Japan also showed chlorella juice has the potential to be a powerful anti-cancer treatment. Lab mice were put on a chlorella regimen for 10 days, and then were injected with three types of cancer. Over 70% of the mice that were fed chlorella didn't develop cancer and 100% of the untreated mice did develop cancer and died within 20 days.

Spirulina is a nutritional supplement with an ancient history of human use. It's cultivated in shallow lakes and used as a dietary supplement, and also in the aquaculture and poultry industries. It was used by the Aztecs, and its sale as cakes was described by one of Hernando Cortez's conquistadors. Spirulina was also used in Chad in Africa as far back as the 9th century Kanem Empire. It's still in daily use there, dried into cakes named *dihe* that are used to make broths for meals.

Spirulina is between 55 and 77% protein by weight. It's a complete protein with all amino acids, except it's lower in methionine, cysteine and lysine than proteins from milk, eggs, or meat. Spirulina protein is superior to all plant proteins, even those from legumes. It's also a rich source of iron, zinc, manganese, chromium, selenium, magnesium, calcium and phosphorus. Spirulina also contains most vitamins in high quantities. There are good reasons why both the Aztecs and the people in Chad in Africa used spirulina for centuries.

SEA SALT

Most health books set up salt as one of the villains in your diet, claiming it is eaten in excess by almost everyone and causes high blood pressure. When you stop eating processed foods, you'll find it's true that less than 4% of the dietary salt consumed in the U.S. comes out of a salt shaker—the rest is listed as ingredients on boxes or cans of 'food.' Lots of research shows high blood pressure is more linked to diets lacking in minerals, such as calcium, potassium, and magnesium, than to salt consumption. Other research shows very low levels of salt are dangerous to your health and put you at risk of heart disease and stroke, indicating salt is important for health. Furthermore, only about 8% of the general population has problems metabolizing salt. If this is you, you're probably aware of it, due to problems with high blood pressure, and have had to be on a salt-restricted diet.

In keeping with the theme of two sides to the same coin, what we do know is that *processed salt* is bad for you, not necessarily real salt. This is understandable when you learn how processed salt is manufactured. In the processing of commercial salt, as many as 85 elements and trace minerals are removed by using chemicals like sulfuric acid, chlorine, and hydrochloric acid. The "salt" is then stripped down to sodium chloride, and iodine is added. The end product is a deadly white, chemical grade of sodium chloride. Processing salt then involves heating it to over 400 degrees and adding anti-caking agents such as ferrocynide, yellow prussiate of soda, tri calcium phosphate, and alumino-calcium silicate or sodium alumino-silicate to keep it free flowing. Up to 2% of chemical additives, such as bleaches, conditioners and anti-caking agents are allowed in commercial salt.

The type of salt you want to consume is naturally harvested sea salt or mineral salts mined from ancient sea beds. When it comes to consuming natural sea salts, our blood plasma and lymph fluids are very similar to the chemical composition of sea water. You start life out in a salty sea of amniotic fluids of your mother's womb, where you grew over three billion times in weight in just nine months. Your cells are adapted to a salty environment, and you need the trace minerals found in the right kind of salts.

A superstar in the world of healthy salts is a natural mineral rock salt mined from ancient sea beds near Richmond, Utah. It has a full complement of beneficial trace minerals. It's a superb product—read about it at www.realsalt.com.

SEA FOOD

I think the statistics are good that eating seafood twice a week cuts the risk of heart disease by 25%. This is a powerful testimony to the vitamins and minerals in seafood, and how nutritious they are to human beings. Like the similar statistics for eating nuts, most likely this phenomena occurs because the American diet is so deficient in trace minerals and adequate vitamins.

However, if you like your seafood, you should do all you can to support groups advocating for clean seas, like the SurfRider Foundation and the Ocean Conservancy. As I write, the world's oceans are undergoing an immense assault on the last remaining maritime resources. There are currently no unexploited or underutilized fisheries anywhere in the world.

The global state of the oceans is a crisis that's equally as pressing as global warming. We live in the wealthiest and most powerful nation in the world, yet we desperately need leadership to help protect and bring back the world's oceans. After global warming, the world's biggest environmental problem is the industrialization of China and the subsequent toxic pollution of the Pacific Ocean. Lax or non-existent environmental regulations allow coal to be burned in Chinese power plants contaminating both the atmosphere and eventually the Pacific Ocean. Toxic metals such as mercury are contaminating both fish and mammals in the Western Pacific Ocean at an escalating pace.

How bad is it? When a killer whale dies in Alaska and washes up on the beach, the state of Alaska now treats that part of the beach as a toxic waste site. Being at the top of the food chain, the whales are concentrating toxins all the time. What will the future hold for our grandchildren, if we don't act now?

The story of the fish known as Chilean Sea Bass and Orange Roughy are harbingers of a dark future where humanity lives on the shores of an ocean without fish. The legendary Chilean Sea Bass is actually a fish called a Patagonian tooth fish that used to be found in large quantities in Antarctic Seas. Aggressive netting of this large, tasty fish caused their prolific numbers to drop precipitously.

But their plight is nothing like that of the Orange Roughy. These populations of a delicious fish with tender white flesh were discovered in large aggregations above deep seamounts off the Southern Australian and Tasmanian coasts. It turns out they *were* a slow-growing, large, deepwater fish that congregated in large schools during mating season. Fishing for them with modern deep water vessels has been the perfect formula for an ecological disaster. Their numbers have dropped dramatically, and they might not recover within your lifetime or mine.

I urge you to try as hard as you can to buy "wild caught" shrimp, fish, and salmon. Worldwide, the epidemic of cheap farm raised fish and shrimp is swamping the markets. However, raising them causes tremendous ecological damage and hurts sustained yield fisheries. Farm raised fish have substantially lower amounts of vital Omega 3 oils than wild caught fish. They're the difference between eating a wild trout caught in cold, fast moving water compared to eating fish fed on Purina Trout Chow in a pond. Viva la difference!

One of the worst environmental horror stories I've heard recently is how poor tribal people in India were being driven from their land by the expanding cultivation of shrimp in coastal ponds. They were pushed further back into the jungles where they were reduced to gathering wild honey from shrinking jungles to support themselves. In their struggles to survive, they were being attacked and eaten by some of the last tigers in India. Ironically, the tigers were probably facing similar challenges of trying to survive in a shrinking habitat. And you think your life is tough?

I'm a strong supporter of efforts to create marine sanctuaries, such as the newly established and highly successful conservation zones at the Channel Islands National Parks off the coast from Santa Barbara, California. This is the last, best hope to bring back healthy populations of wildlife by closing down both commercial and sport harvesting of seafood. It's believed that the healthy populations of lobsters, fish, crabs, scallops, and abalones in larval form will re-seed and repopulate the adjoining areas. The story is just beginning and it's already becoming a huge success story. It's one that needs to be replicated in other areas of the U.S.

Adopting practices of sustained yield of resources is the only future for the world's oceans. The high seas are truly the last frontier. We've reached the ends of exploitation and have to change....or die. If you want to make a difference, I suggest you join the Ocean Conservancy and the Surf Rider Foundation. They can be reached online at www. oceanconservancy.org or www.surfrider.org.

In the last chapter of this book, I've given you the ultimate Channel Islands abalone recipe. My last comment about the sad state of the fisheries in Southern California is: Bring back the abalone!

BUTTER

As I mentioned earlier, when I started out on this health quest, I was confused about what's good for you and what was bad. I started out eliminating butter and trying to eat it as little as possible. I, like most 21st century Americans, thought it was a devilish product created by cloven hoofed cows, designed to make you fat and plug your arteries with cholesterol sludge.

You read in this chapter about how eating avocados with your salad causes your body to greatly increase your absorption of vitamins—the same story is true for butter. Eating butter or olive oil with Swiss chard, asparagus, green beans, snap peas, beets, etc. will greatly increase your absorption of vitamins. Butter—a health food? Surprisingly enough, this is the truth. Try to find a good source of butter that comes from cows grazing in green pastures. The highest caliber butter is the earliest butter that's deep orange colored and comes from cows eating the first grasses of springtime.

I've come full circle from trying to devise recipes for making tofu tasty, to drinking raw milk and eating butter from cows grazing in the green pastures of Wisconsin. Who would ever think, after all the brainwashing we've come through, that I'd be extolling the virtues of butter as a health food? Eat butter—its real food—and good for you!

Best Foods For a Hospital Stay

I want to end this chapter with a recommendation for the kind of foods you need to be eating if you are recovering from illness or injury in a hospital. If you ever find yourself in a hospital and you know anything about healthy foods and natural healing, you'll realize eating American hospital food is one of the worst things you can possibly do. The cafeteria style food in most hospitals comes from standard industrial food sources containing industrial dairy, industrial chicken, industrial meat, and other processed foods lacking in nutrients. The menu, made usually of generic American foods, is high in dangerous polyunsaturated (vegetable) oils and full of sugar, hydrogenated oils, oxidized cholesterols, and corn syrup. This is what your body is going to use as fuel to help you heal?

The following nutritional Rx is made up of the sort of foods you should be eating to heal yourself if you're in a hospital. This nutritional regimen was devised by Dr. Weston Price, the dentist and pioneer of nutritional health from Cleveland, and was used to drastically improve the health of children living in a group home in the latter years of the Great Depression. Price monitored the children's dental and physical health closely, and his records show this diet worked wonders for them.

Here's a description of what the children ate before Dr. Price introduced his regimen, and what they ate after the supplemental elements of the regiment, as quoted from his book, *Nutrition and Physical Degeneration*, published in 1939.

It was important to note that the home diet which had been responsible for the tooth decay was exceedingly low in body building and repair material and high in sweets and refined starches. It usually consisted of a highly sweetened coffee and white bread, vegetable fat, pancakes made of white flour and eaten with syrup and donuts fried in vegetable fat.

The diet provided these children in the supplemental meal was as follows: About four ounces of tomato juice or orange juice and a teaspoonful of a mixture of equal parts of a very high vitamin, natural cod liver oil and an especially high vitamin butter oil was given at the beginning of the meal. The child then received a bowl containing approximately a pint of a very rich vegetable and meat stew, made largely from bone marrow and fine cuts of tender meat. The meat was usually broiled separately to retain its juice and then chopped very fine and added to the bone marrow meat soup, which always contained finely chopped vegetables and plenty of little yellow carrots. The next course consisted of cooked fruit, with very little sweetening, and rolls made from freshly ground whole wheat and spread with high vitamin butter. The wheat for the rolls was ground fresh every day in a motor-driven coffee mill. Each child was given also two glasses of fresh whole milk. The menu was varied from day to day by substituting for the meat stew, fish chowder or organs of animals."

Now that's not exactly what you expect to see on the tray brought in by the nurse at dinnertime, is it? Better to reach for the phone and call a friend or family member to bring you some real food if you ever want to get out of that hospital!

⌐

One of my biggest complaints with most diet and health books is that they offer terribly boring recipes. Who wants to eat boring food? Being healthy doesn't have to be boring.

In the next and final chapter, I hope to entice you into eating more of the foods that are good for you and for your waistline by providing a collection of recipes I myself have used in my own kitchen. I find them unique, fun and tasty. I hope you enjoy these recipes, and they help you eat food that tastes good and is good for you.

CHAPTER TWELVE

The Santa Barbara Long Life Diet— Recipes For A Better World

Many years ago, I would never have dreamed of titling a book *The Santa Barbara Diet*. Back then, I didn't want the rest of the world to know about our beautiful town of Santa Barbara. But those days are long gone, and we don't have any choice but to share our Santa Barbara with the rest of the world. It seems hard to believe it was once a sleepy little beach town with only a few restaurants that stayed open after the sun went down. It seems like only yesterday…

Recently, I had the pleasure of sitting in the home of a long-time Santa Barbara local who, with his wife, built their home on a hillside overlooking the Old Mission. Now in his nineties, my friend told me that when he was a boy, he lived down the street from his current home, and until World War II, the *padres*—Spanish priests who lived at the Old Mission—kept their cattle penned up where now there were open lawns. As a boy, he and his brother kept their horses in a large corral that is now replaced by the City Rose Gardens across from the Old Mission.

With a gleam in his eye he told me how when they were children, they'd ride their horses all over Santa Barbara. Some days he'd walk up the hillside beyond the horse pen into a grove of pine tress and sit and read books on a small hill overlooking the Old Mission. Much later in life, he and his wife built their dream house on the same location, where I sat with them in their living room enjoying the view of the Old Mission.

I'm giving you this perspective because I'd like you, too, to live to be almost 90 years old, like these Santa Barbara natives, and live in your own home and not need anyone to care for you. Much that is involved in living a long life we have little control over, but making healthy and smart choices in our diet is something we can control. That's what the following simple recipes for healthy living are all about.

An Evolving Cuisine

In the old days, long before the explosion of "new wave," Santa Barbara style cooking, the locals were experts at barbecuing tri-tip steaks, grilling white sea bass, halibut and abalone, eating locally grown vegetables and fruits, and enjoying pinquito beans and Lima beans grown in the sandy soils near Carpinteria.

Even if you're from Santa Barbara, you may not have known that the town of Carpinteria was named by the Spanish Conquistadores almost 400 years ago. They came down the coastline wearing hats and breastplates made of steel, and discovered the natives building unique planked boats from the redwood logs that had washed up on the sandy beaches of the Central Coast. They named the place *Carpinteria*, which means "wood-shop." The Chumash Indians used to travel in their big sea-going canoes up and down the coast and out to the offshore islands, and I'm sure they usually returned with large quantities of the abundant abalones, lobsters, scallops, mussels, halibut, swordfish, and rockfish available at that time.

Santa Barbara is still a timeless place, and our cuisine reflects the many peoples who have inhabited this special area. Now the local cuisine is a blend of Mediterranean, Italian, Basque, French, and Asian foods, and, of course, food from old Mexico. I wrote most of this book in Santa Barbara, so I have to admit, I've been under the magic spell that the *City by the Sea* casts upon you. Time has always stood still for me in Santa Barbara, and I try to appreciate every day as much as I can. Who knows what tomorrow will bring?

A glance at the restaurant offerings in Santa Barbara on a recent Valentine's Day is a good indicator of Santa Barbara style cuisine. How about some cilantro-crusted sea bass with lobster red curry sauce and sweet potato ravioli? Or braised short rib tortellini with parsley and oven-roasted tomato and pine nut crème? The choices go on to include grilled Moorish-spiced venison, or heart-shaped scallop ravioli with lobster sauce, or Dungeness crabmeat and jumbo prawns.....

Here in Santa Barbara, we're incredibly fortunate to have our Farmers' Market that has to be one of the best farmers' markets in the world. It certainly encourages you to make your own fresh squeezed orange juice when you can buy a 25 pound bag of Valencia oranges for as little as $7. My mother, Mary (age 81 and going strong), loves to shop at the Farmers' Market as much as anyone else in Santa Barbara. Even if you have your own garden or fruit trees, you would need to have a huge rancho and a lot of help to duplicate the experience available almost every day of the week in different locations in and around Santa Barbara.

Smoked garlic, Santa Maria strawberries, ridgeback shrimp, walnut oil, medjhool dates, Lemon Quark cheese, lobsters from Anacapa Island, jojoba oil, parsnips, tangerines, heirloom tomatoes, deepwater oysters from offshore Hope Ranch, sweet corn, and the last fresh peaches in October—these are just some of the foods I see in the downtown Market on a typical Saturday morning. We're a lucky bunch living here and enjoying the fruits of the earth. But wherever you live, be sure you do all you can to support your local growers and fisher folks!

Of course, we can also shop in a lot of wonderful, healthy food stores in Santa Barbara and environs, including the gourmet Lazy Acres, the ubiquitous Trader Joe's (three of them!), and the Indo-Pacific Market in Goleta. It wouldn't be fair not mentioning our own local handmade ice cream store, McConnell's, along with the wharf-side Fisherman's Market that opens early Saturday morning, the Italian deli Via Maestra, and soon—a Whole Foods supermarket (Good luck making it in Santa Barbara!), and all of the other myriad food establishments that help consummate the culinary experience of the seriously committed food experts who live in Santa Barbara, California.

For times when you're feasting and not fasting, I thought I'd recommend a few places in old Santa Barbara—the Santa Barbara I've known for so many decades. One of my favorites for a simple breakfast is the Xanadu Café in Montecito. It's the best bakery in town and is open seven days a week, starting at 4:30 am. This is the place to eat if you're on the way to the harbor to get an early start heading up the Channel to San Miguel Island or before going to Rincon Point to paddle your board out to meet the rising sun and beat the crowds.

Of course, you wouldn't want to leave Santa Barbara without eating lunch at Norton's Pastrami on Figueroa in the hustling heart of the central business district. And don't miss eating *sopes* and *tacos* made from freshly prepared corn tortillas at La Super Rica Taqueria, unquestionably the best and most original Mexican food in town. A drive up Milpas Street never fails to show the line of natives and visitors winding around the corner patiently waiting for a chance to order and sit in the open air café. The best Mexican food in California? I'll leave the verdict up to you....

We certainly have our indulgences here in Santa Barbara, and we don't need help finding delicious food. But therein lies the seeds of the Santa Barbara Diet that you've been reading about in this book. If you love good food and you always have an abundance of it, learning how to do nutritionally assisted fasting is a necessity in order to stay healthy and keep excess weight off. Fasting helps us Santa Barbarans to control our native proclivities for enjoying this ongoing feast, and fasting can allow you to enjoy eating the food you love and still maintain your health and perfect weight.

Enjoying and appreciating good homemade and handmade food is one of the joys of life, but being overweight is a curse. I'm about to introduce you to many good recipes, and even though they're made from natural and healthy ingredients—if you eat too much of anything— you'll have trouble controlling your weight. Learning how to fast (See Chapter 9) and understanding how little food your body truly needs to survive helps us to control our natural tendency of enjoying too much of a good thing.

Santa Barbara Lifestyle

I'd be remiss in not taking time to make a few comments about the habits of the Santa Barbara natives. So far, I've been as politically correct as someone like me can be, but I can't help but comment on a few of the habits of the natives.

One of the hallmarks of the Santa Barbara style is always being late for everything. Showing up on time is either *gauche, passé,* or simply clueless—you choose which. In Santa Barbara, being 15 minutes late is "spot on"—*a punto*—as they say in Old Mexico. There's a sense of timelessness in Santa Barbara, yet at the same time, you can't help but realize how quickly everything passes when you're standing beneath the mountains at the edge of the Pacific Ocean. Where else but in Santa Barbara would you change your route homeward to enjoy a better view of the setting sun?

At the same time, nothing could be more "Santa Barbara" than fleeing because the seasonal fog is getting on your nerves. Out to the desert or off to the South Pacific—it must be better somewhere else when the thick layers of fog start moving in and take away our sunshine. Isn't it supposed to be sunny and perfect, everyday in Santa Barbara? You've got a bad case of *Santa Barbara Syndrome* when you expect both the weather and life to be perfect all the time. This tendency of the natives is almost as deeply genetically coded as another tendency of being *Santa Barbara Nice*....often, *too* nice, to mix well in other crueler locales in a tumultuous world.

Santa Barbara is a locale where even the most hyperactive, compulsive business men get stopped in their tracks by the sacred beauty of each fleeting minute as it pulses beneath the warm California sun. Sometimes it takes a few acerbic comments from outsiders like newspaper columnist Ashleigh Brilliant (he wasn't born here), to make us realize the truth about our sleepy little town. In his syndicated column, *Pot-Shots*, he once penned the immortal words: *Nothing important ever happens in Santa Barbara.* I'm sure Mary Miles Minter, Marilyn Monroe, and John Kennedy thought what they did in Santa Barbara was of paramount importance, but the rest of us mortals who live here might not be so convinced.

Unfortunately, you may not be able to take Santa Barbara with you wherever you go in life, but you can take these simple recipes with you and the joy of living under a warm sun where the good things in life are alive and well....

SANTA BARBARA RECIPES FOR A BETTER WORLD

I hope you enjoy these recipes—most of them are designed with your health in mind and use simple, natural ingredients to help you develop new ways of cooking vegetables, grains, fish, fruits, meats and fowl. In contrast to the average recipes you find in a typical American cookbook, the emphasis here is on good health and good nutrition. Anyone can cook food that tastes good but isn't good for you. These recipes attempt to accomplish the opposite: food that tastes good and is good for you.

That being said, I highly recommend you only use the freshest, organic, unprocessed foods available to you when preparing these recipes. Always choose raw dairy products, grass-fed meats, free-range chickens and eggs, and the host of other truly natural and highly nutritious foods you have been introduced to throughout this book. In regards to oils, use vegetable oils that are not rancid or hydrogenated, such as grapeseed, walnut, sesame, and peanut. Stay away from cheap margarines, soybean oils, partially hydrogenated or hydrogenated vegetable oils and oils like Wesson oil, which is made from cheap blends of soybean and cottonseed oils.

Here's to your enjoyment! May you enjoy the blessings of good health and a long life.....

Vegetables & Grains

Roasted Roma Tomatoes

Roma tomatoes are the best for roasting because they have the lowest moisture content of tomatoes. They're good to eat hot or cold, chopped and tossed with salads, or pureed and added to sauces to enhance the flavor.

INGREDIENTS: 8 large Roma tomatoes
½ Teaspoon of Real Salt or sea salt
¼ cup olive oil

PREPARATION: Preheat oven to 350 degrees. Wash and dry tomatoes.

1. Cut tomatoes in half, lengthwise and place in a large bowl. Season with salt, sprinkle lightly with pepper and toss with olive oil.
2. Place cut side up on a large baking sheet. Roast them on the top rack of your oven for about one hour or until caramelized. Serve hot from the oven or cool slightly. *Enjoy!*

Sweet Potato Wedges with Parmesan and Yoghurt Aioli

INGREDIENTS: 6 medium sweet potatoes
2 Tablespoons olive oil
2 Tablespoons coconut oil
2 Tablespoons Parmesan cheese
1 Teaspoon salt
1 Teaspoon pepper

YOGHURT AIOLI: ½ cup plain yoghurt
2 Tablespoons mayonnaise
1 Tablespoon lemon juice
2 cloves of finely minced garlic
Salt and pepper to taste

PREPARATION:

1. Preheat oven to 400 degrees. Cut sweet potatoes into half inch wedges.
2. Put the cut potatoes in a bowl and sprinkle with olive oil, coconut oil, salt and pepper, and toss well.
3. Lay out potatoes on a baking sheet.
4. Roast for 45 minutes, and halfway through baking, remove from oven and stir them. Watch closely after 30 minutes. Turn down heat, if needed.
5. When almost done, sprinkle Parmesan cheese liberally over the wedges and return to the oven for 5 minutes.
6. Mix all ingredients for Yoghurt Aioli together and serve with warm potatoes.

Sunland Salad

INGREDIENTS: 2 perfect navel oranges
2 ripe Haas avocados
1 large sweet onion, Maui, Walla Walla or Vidalia
Oil and vinegar dressing
2 Tablespoons finely minced green onion

PREPARATION:

1. Peel oranges, remove white pith and slice thinly.
2. Peel and slice avocados.
3. Cut onion into thin slices.
4. On a glass plate or fine China, arrange rings of alternating, overlapping slices of oranges, avocados, and onions. Drizzle with dressing.
5. Garnish with green onions and chill before serving.

Honey-Butter Carrots

INGREDIENTS: 1 pound of scraped and thinly sliced carrots
2 Tablespoons of butter
2 Tablespoons of honey

PREPARATION:

1. Prepare carrots and cook in boiling, salted water uncovered, about 5 minutes or until barely cooked.
2. Remove from boiling water and set aside to drain.
3. In medium size sauce pan on medium to high heat, melt butter and sauté carrots for 1 to 2 minutes to glaze them.

Curried Root Vegetables

INGREDIENTS: 2 Tablespoons of coconut oil or olive oil
1 or 2 cloves of minced garlic
1 small onion cut into small pieces
2 to 3 Teaspoons of curry powder
3 medium carrots
1 yam
1 potato
3 tomatoes, roughly chopped

1 cup tomato juice
Salt and pepper

PREPARATION:

1. In a large pot, warm over medium low heat.
2. Add garlic and onions and sauté until tender. Add curry powder and mustard seeds. Cook for 2 or 3 minutes.
3. Peel carrots, yams, and potato and slice into one inch chunks. Add to onions and garlic mixture. Add tomatoes and tomato juice.
4. Put lid on and cook on low heat for 20 to 25 minutes or until veggies are tender. Season with salt and pepper.

Roasted Winter Root Vegetables with Horseradish Yoghurt Sauce

INGREDIENTS:	2 medium red onions
2 medium parsnips, peeled
1 medium rutabaga, peeled
1 medium celery root (celeriac), peeled
1 teaspoon butter
1 teaspoon olive oil
2 Tablespoons coconut oil or olive oil
1 head garlic
Lemon wedges

HORSERADISH YOGHURT SAUCE:

2 Teaspoons horseradish
2/3 cup plain yoghurt
Juice of ½ lemon
Salt and freshly ground pepper

PREPARATION:

1. Preheat oven to 400 degrees. Bring large pot of water to roiling boil.
2. Trim tops of onions and peel outer skin without removing root. Cut into quarters, leaving root attached. Cut all other veggies into one inch chunks.
3. Mix oils and warmed butter in small bowl and put into roasting pan and warm in oven. Place vegetables in boiling water and boil for 5 minutes. Drain vegetables and place them in sizzling butter and oils. Turn so they're oiled on all sides.
4. Bake uncovered for 15 minutes. Break garlic into individual cloves but don't peel. Add garlic to the veggies and roast for 20 minutes or until they're golden brown and tender.
5. Sauce: While vegetables are roasting, prepare sauce. Mix together horseradish, sour cream, lemon juice and seasonings and chill until needed.
6. Serve vegetables on large platter with lemon wedges and the sauce.

Quinoa Hot Pot

INGREDIENTS:

2 Tablespoons butter
2 Tablespoons of coconut oil
4 shallots or one large onion, peeled and chopped
2 cloves of finely minced garlic-use smoked garlic if you have it.
1 stalk of celery, finely chopped
2 medium carrots, chopped
2 fresh tomatoes, chopped
1 cup of quinoa, well rinsed
1 Teaspoon of garam Marsala
2 cups of homemade chicken stock (Use a quality brand such as Swenson's, if you don't have homemade.)
¼ cup minced fresh parsley

PREPARATION:

1. Melt butter and coconut oil.
2. Add shallots, garlic, celery and carrots and sauté for 3 to 5 minutes or until veggies are soft.
3. Add chopped tomatoes and quinoa.
4. Cook for a few minutes—then add stock.
5. Season with salt and pepper, bring to a boil, then turn heat down to low.
6. Cover and simmer for about 45 minutes.
7. Uncover, add garam Marsala and chopped parsley, and cook for another 5 minutes.

Cranberry Couscous

INGREDIENTS:

1 Tablespoon of butter
1 Tablespoon of coconut oil
1 cup finely chopped onion
1 clove, finely minced garlic
½ cup dried cranberries
2 Teaspoons of lemon zest
12 oz. of couscous (Buy the large style Israeli couscous if you can)
1 Teaspoon of salt
2 cups of chicken stock (boiling)
4 Tablespoons, chopped parsley

PREPARATION:

1. Melt butter and coconut oil in large frying pan over medium heat. Sauté onion and

garlic until transparent, being careful not to burn them.

2. Add couscous, lemon zest, cranberries, salt, and boiling liquid. Mix together and pour mixture into a 6 cup Pyrex baking dish.

3. Cover dish and bake at 375 for 15 minutes. Remove from oven and fluff with fork. Sprinkle with chopped parsley.

C

Swiss Chard Pie

INGREDIENTS: 1 lb. of chard, washed, trimmed and finely chopped.

2 Tablespoons of fresh chopped herbs (basil, thyme, rosemary, parsley, cilantro, etc.)

1 red onion, chopped

2 Tablespoons of olive oil

6 eggs

1 cup of grated cheese

2/3 cup of half and half

Pie crust: Makes 1 pie top and bottom crust; 9 inch size in a deep Pyrex dish.

¾ cups of King Arthur bleached all purpose flour

¾ cups of King Arthur white whole wheat flour

1 Tsp. of Real Salt

½ cup of butter (Use Kerry Gold or Double Devon Cream butter from Trader Joe's or your local health food store.)

A little less than 1/3 cup of water

PREPARATION FOR PIE CRUST:

1. Cut butter into small pieces and add slowly to well sifted flour and salt mixture.
2. Cut butter in with dough mixer tool or use fork.
3. Gradually add water, and mix until just barely mixed.
4. Work dough as little as possible to blend it. Use as little water as possible.
5. Add carefully, bit by bit, to make sure you don't get it too wet. Roll into ball and place in refrigerator and chill for 15 minutes.
6. Cut dough in half and roll half out and line pie pan.

PREPARATION:

7. Add olive oil to large sauté pan and cook red onion until tender. Then add chard and sauté until well softened then add herbs.
8. Turn the oven to 350 degrees and mix beaten eggs, half and half, and cheese in a large bowl.
9. Put pie crust in pie pan and trim edges.
10. Put chard and onion mixture in pie pan and pour eggs & cheese mixture over the top.
11. Make pie crust with remaining half of dough (lattice top is best) and put over mixture and seal edges.
12. Bake for 45 minutes or until filling is firm and crust is golden brown.

Fava Bean Gratin

My friend, Manuel Josta, who immigrated to Santa Barbara from the Azore Islands, used to grow fava beans in a garden plot on the top of a hill in Goleta. Manuel had the greenest thumb of any human being I've ever met. I loved his address: La Buena Tierra, (The Good Earth) Goleta, California, USA. It was many years later when I saw these beans in the Farmer's Market downtown and finally learned how to cook them. I quickly learned why the folks from the Old Country liked them so much.

INGREDIENTS: 6 pounds fresh fava beans in the pod (This makes about 3 ½ cups shelled and peeled beans)

3 Tablespoons unsalted butter

3 Large shallots, finely chopped

¾ Teaspoon *Real Salt* or sea salt

¼ Teaspoon finely ground white pepper

4 Tablespoons, freshly chopped parsley

2 Tablespoons, finely ground, dried bread crumbs

4 Tablespoons freshly grated sheep's milk cheese or Parmesan cheese

PREPARATION:

1. Shell the fava beans.
2. Fill a large saucepan, 2/3rds full of water, and bring to a roiling boil.
3. Add beans to boiling water and blanch until tender (2 or 3 minutes). Drain, and pinch off the skins with your fingers and set aside.
4. Pre-heat broiler.
5. Warm butter and shallots in sauté pan with medium heat and sauté until shallots are clear (2 or 3 minutes). Add fava beans, pepper, salt, and parsley and stir gently. Cook for 2 or 3 more minutes.
6. Transfer mixture to shallow, ovenproof serving dish. Put breadcrumbs and cheese evenly over the top. Place under broiler until surface is lightly browned, about 3 to 5 minutes.

Braised Fennel in Orange Juice and White Wine with Thyme

INGREDIENTS: 3 medium size fennel bulbs trimmed and cut in half. Save fronds.

3 Tablespoons of olive oil

¼ cup dry white wine

5 cloves of garlic, chopped

¾ cup freshly squeezed orange juice

1 Tablespoon fresh thyme

PREPARATION:

1. Rub the fennel halves with 2 Tablespoons of olive oil and season with salt and pepper.
2. Put 1 Tablespoon of olive oil in large skillet over high heat. Add fennel and cook with cut side down for about 5 minutes, or until golden brown color. Flip over and cook other side for about 3 minutes.
3. Pour in wine and bring to a boil, wait 30 seconds, then add garlic, orange juice, and thyme.
4. Bring to a boil again, then cover pan and turn heat down to medium low. Simmer until fennel is tender (about 8 to 10 minutes).
5. Uncover and cook over medium heat until pan juices are reduced, about 10 minutes.
6. Serve warm and sprinkle with chopped fronds.

Spinach Salad with Caramelized Onions, Poached Eggs and Crispy Prosciutto

This dish serves four fortunate souls. . . .

INGREDIENTS: 1 Tablespoon plus 1 Teaspoon of olive oil

1 Tablespoon unsalted butter

1 large red onion, sliced very thin

1 Tablespoon of honey

4 ounces of thinly sliced Prosciutto, cut into one inch pieces

6 cups fresh spinach

¼ cup Vinaigrette (see following recipe)

4 large poached eggs (see following recipe)

Salt and freshly ground pepper

PREPARATION:

1. In sauté pan, heat butter and one teaspoon of oil over medium heat. Add onion, cook for 4 minutes or until translucent colored. Add honey, cook one more minute or until onion is golden brown. Remove from pan to cool down.

2. Heat remaining Tablespoon of oil and add Prosciutto pieces. Cook for about one minute, then flip them over and cook until other side is crispy, about four minutes. Remove to paper towels to drain.

3. Place spinach in large salad bowl. Add onion and Prosciutto.
Toss well with prepared vinaigrette. Divide salad and place on four plates. Place poached egg on top of each serving and sprinkle with salt and pepper.

VINAIGRETTE:	2 Tablespoons of minced shallots
	1 Tablespoon Dijon style mustard
	¼ red wine vinegar or aged rice wine vinegar
	½ cup olive oil
	Whisk all ingredients together in a large measuring cup except the olive oil. Add olive oil slowly and mix until it's well blended. You can make vinaigrette in advance and keep in refrigerator.

POACHED EGGS:

4. Boil 8 cups of water in a large pan, add a pinch of salt and 1 Tablespoon of rice wine vinegar.

5. Crack one egg into small bowl. Slide egg carefully into pan and boil for two minutes, or until done. Skim off foam.

6. Use slotted spoon to transfer egg to a plate to drain. Pat gently with paper towel. Repeat with remaining eggs.

c̓

Balsamic Sweet Potato Fries

INGREDIENTS:	2 pounds of sweet potatoes, cut into 3 to 4 inch French fries
	4 Tablespoons of coconut oil
	½ Teaspoon of paprika
	¼ Teaspoon of *Real Salt* or sea salt
	1 Tablespoon of aged balsamic vinegar
	Cooking spray (Use olive oil instead of canola—it's better for you.)

PREPARATION:

1. Preheat oven to 400 degrees. Coat baking sheet with cooking spray.
2. Toss sweet potato fries with coconut oil, paprika, salt, and pepper.
3. Place fries in one layer on baking sheet and bake for 25 to 30 minutes. Watch closely after 20 minutes, so they don't burn or stick.
4. Remove from oven, sprinkle with balsamic vinegar and toss to coat.

c̓

Kabocha Squash

If you've never tried these delicious squashes grown on the Central California coast, you have a real taste treat in store. Kabochas are a heirloom variety of pumpkin from Japan with high levels of beta-carotene and sugars. The orange variety, Sunshine Kabocha, has a very thin skin that is edible. They're excellent filling for healthy pumpkin pies, too. They keep in storage for up to three months.

INGREDIENTS: 1 large Kabocha Squash

PREPARATION:

1. Bake whole in the oven. Scrub very well, then poke a vent hole in it with a knife, put on oven rack and bake at 400 degrees for one hour.
2. Let cool a few minutes, then cut in half and remove seeds.
3. Enjoy!

Stir Fried Greens

Italian Style —

PREPARATION:

1. Cut chard, spinach, kale or cabbage leaves into ¾ inch strips.
2. Heat olive oil in large pan and sauté finely minced garlic.
3. When almost done add flavored vinaigrette or a small amount of aged balsamic vinegar.
4. Sprinkle with lemon juice and serve topped with toasted pistachio nuts.

Eastern European Style —

PREPARATION:

1. Cut kale or cabbage leaves into ¾ inch strips.
2. Season with olive oil and butter and season with caraway and salt and pepper.

Asian Style —

PREPARATION:

1. Cut Bok Choy, Guy Lon, Napa cabbage or baby Bok Choy into ¾ inch pieces.
2. Stir fry in sesame or peanut oil.
3. Season with garlic, ginger, soy sauce, rice wine vinegar or lime juice.

Santa Barbara Style Guacamole

INGREDIENTS:

5 medium Hass avocados
3 Tablespoons of lime juice
¼ cup salsa
1 medium size onion, chopped finely
2 cloves of garlic, finely minced
1 Teaspoon of salt
1 Teaspoon of black pepper
1 Teaspoon of cumin
3 chopped roma tomatoes or one large tomato
1 cup of finely chopped cilantro
2 chopped green onions
1 Tablespoon of coconut oil

PREPARATION:

1. Sauté garlic and onion in coconut oil
2. Remove from heat and cool.
3. Chop avocados, add all other ingredients and mix well
4. Taste and adjust all seasonings.

Curried Lentil Spread

INGREDIENTS:

8 ounces of orange lentils. (Soak in water for 12 hours and sprout for 36 to 48 hours by spreading in a pie tin and rinsing twice daily until well-sprouted. As an alternative, you can cook ½ pound of lentils by covering with water and simmering for 30 minutes.)
2 Tablespoons of coconut oil
1 medium onion, finely chopped
1 finely chopped garlic clove
3 Teaspoons of curry powder
6 marinated or dried tomatoes. (Soak in hot water to re-constitute, if they're not packed in oil.)
2 Teaspoons of lemon juice
½ Teaspoon black pepper
Salt to taste

PREPARATION:

1. Heat coconut oil and sauté onions and garlic. Mix in curry powder and cook thoroughly.
2. Put lentils in processor and add cooked, spiced onions.
3. Add all other ingredients and blend until smooth.
4. Serve on crackers, romaine lettuce wraps, or use as a dip for cut vegetables.

⚬

Living Hummus

INGREDIENTS:
1 cup of dried garbanzo beans
2 cloves of finely minced garlic
1 seeded jalapeno pepper
2 chopped green onions
½ cup olive oil
1/3 cup lemon juice
3 Tablespoons of miso
3 Tablespoons of tahini (sesame butter or paste)
Optional: sun dried tomatoes, capers, fresh tomatoes, celery, chopped fresh peppers, etc.

PREPARATION:

1. Soak one cup of dried garbanzo beans in a bowl of cold water for 12 hours. Drain, cover with a paper towel, and sprout beans for 24 to 48 hours.
2. Rinse them twice a day with pure water and keep them moist.
3. Combine in a food processor with garlic, jalapeno, and chopped green onions.
4. Add olive oil, lemon juice, tahini and miso.
5. Eat on crispy lettuce leaves, Middle Eastern Lavash bread or on small triangles of whole wheat pita bread.

⚬

Quinoa Stuffed Peppers

INGREDIENTS:
1 cup of quinoa
2 cups of chicken stock or water
6 to 8 medium yellow, red, or green peppers
1 medium onion diced
½ pound fresh mushrooms, sliced
2 Tablespoons coconut oil
1 28 ounce can of tomatoes, coarsely diced (save the juice)
2 crushed garlic cloves
2 Tablespoons dry sherry
6 ounces of mozzarella cheese, shredded

PREPARATION:

1. Place quinoa and water or chicken stock in 1 ½ quart saucepan and bring to a boil. Reduce to a simmer and cook until water is absorbed, about 10 to 15 minutes.
2. Cut tops from peppers, clean seeds and cut ribs out.
3. Steam peppers in a large pan with a small amount of water until soft, but not totally limp.

4. In a large skillet, sauté onion, garlic and mushrooms in coconut oil. Add diced tomatoes and Mexican salsa.
5. Reserve 4 or 5 Tablespoons of salsa.
6. Cook over medium heat for five minutes. Add sherry and simmer for five more minutes. Fold in quinoa and stir well.
7. Place peppers in baking dish and fill with quinoa.
8. Pour in reserved juice from can around peppers and top peppers with reserved salsa and mozzarella.
9. Bake in 325 degree oven for 30 minutes.

Soups

Beef, Barley and Mushroom Soup

This soup freezes well, and canned or fresh tomatoes are a good addition.

INGREDIENTS:
1 ounce dried shitake mushrooms, soaked in two cups boiling water for 30 minutes.
2 Tablespoons olive oil
3 leeks, white and light green parts only, cleaned and coarsely chopped
2 beef shanks, salt and freshly ground black pepper
½ cup pearl barley
2 carrots, peeled and coarsely chopped
1 pound white button mushrooms
7 cups of beef or chicken broth
1 Tablespoon of soy sauce
3 Tablespoons finely chopped parsley

PREPARATION:

1. Strain dried mushrooms over a bowl, squeeze dry and save one cup of the soaking liquid. Dice mushrooms into ¼ inch pieces and put in a small bowl.
2. Strain reserved soaking liquid and pour through sieve onto mushrooms.
3. In a large pot, heat olive oil over medium high heat. Add leeks and sauté 5 to 7 minutes, until softened. Season the beef shanks with salt and pepper and add to the leeks. Brown them on each side for about 2 minutes.
4. Add barley, fresh mushrooms, carrots and sauté until coated—about one minute. Add the broth, reduce heat to low, cover and simmer for 1 to 1 ½ hours or until barley is tender.
5. Remove the beef and let it cool. Shred the meat and return it to the soup. Add the reserved dried mushroom mixture to the soup. Add soy sauce and parsley and simmer for five minutes or so. Season with salt and pepper and serve immediately.

White Bean and Potato Soup with Olive Puree

INGREDIENTS:
½ cup olive oil or rendered duck fat
1 medium onion, sliced into thick slices
6 garlic cloves, crushed
1 sprig fresh rosemary
2 small russet potatoes (about ½ pound)
2 cups dried white beans, soaked for 8 to 10 hours in water
10 cups Vegetable Stock, preferably homemade
1 Tablespoon *Real Salt* or sea salt
¼ Teaspoon freshly ground white pepper
25 pitted, green Spanish olives or Greek Kalamata olives

PREPARATION:

1. Warm olive oil over high heat in a large pan with a thick bottom. Add onion, garlic, and rosemary and sauté for 5 minutes.
2. Rinse beans under cold running water in a colander.
3. Add beans, potatoes, vegetable stock and salt and pepper in stock pot and bring to a boil. Reduce heat to a simmer, and cook, covered for one hour or until beans are tender. Remove rosemary and season with salt and pepper *al gusto*.
4. Put soup in a blender or food processor and puree on high speed for one minute. Return soup to saucepan and bring to a boil.
5. Puree olives in food processor and mix until pureed. Put pureed olives into squeeze bottle or plastic bag with corner cut off with scissors.
6. Ladle bean soup into bowls and garnish by squeezing pureed olive in swirls on each portion.

Portuguese Caldo Verde (Green Soup)

INGREDIENTS:
1 large bunch of kale, washed and trimmed, and cut into very thin strips
1/3 cup of white beans, soaked overnight
½ cup olive oil
3 quarts chicken stock
3 medium onions, sliced very thin
2 to 3 large potatoes, peeled and grated
3 large cloves of garlic, minced
1 Bay Leaf
½ pound of Italian sausage, cut into ½ slices (optional)

PREPARATION:

1. In a large stockpot, heat the olive oil and sauté garlic, onions, and sausage.
2. Add the kale, beans, chicken stock, and potatoes.

3. Bring to a boil, and then simmer for 2 hours with cover on.
4. Salt and pepper to taste.
5. Serve with a green salad and baguettes.

Hmong Market Soup

This is a different soup with a hot and spicy, sour flavor. Just the thing to savor as you watch the fisherman set their nets for the elusive giant catfish on the Mekong River in the golden dusk at a sidewalk café in Luang Prabang in Laos.....

INGREDIENTS
½ onion, peeled and chopped
1 carrot, cut into thin matchstick pieces
2 Tablespoons dark sesame oil
1 clove of garlic, peeled and crushed
1 Tablespoon of shredded fresh gingerroot
1 stalk of lemon grass or one Tablespoon of fresh lemon juice
2 cups of homemade chicken stock
3 cups of canned coconut milk
2 Tablespoons of peanut butter
1 cup of shredded, cooked chicken meat
Salt and fresh ground pepper to taste
½ Teaspoon of turmeric or one inch piece of turmeric, well shredded
½ Teaspoon of red pepper flakes
¼ cup of chopped fresh cilantro for garnish

PREPARATION:

1. In a large saucepan, cook onion and carrot in sesame oil until tender. In a blender or food processor, puree garlic, ginger, lemongrass stalk, stock and coconut milk.
2. Pour into large pot, add sautéed vegetables and bring to a simmer.
3. In a small cup, mix peanut butter and ¼ cup of hot soup, then pour back into pot.
4. Add cooked chicken, salt, pepper, turmeric and red pepper.
5. Serve immediately and garnish with lime slice and cilantro.

Food for Entertaining

Baked Pasta with Italian Sausage and Spicy Tomato Sauce

This recipe serves 6 to 8—or double the recipe and freeze half for later use.

INGREDIENTS:
- 1 pound hot Italian sausage with casings removed
- 1 large onion, finely chopped
- 3 minced garlic cloves
- 2-26 ounce cans of good marinara sauce
- 6 Tablespoons of basil pesto
- Salt and freshly ground black pepper
- 1 pound of penne pasta
- ½ pound smoked Gouda or mozzarella cheese, finely grated
- 1 cup freshly grated Parmesan cheese
- 1-6 ounce bag of baby spinach leaves, or use more, if you like.

PREPARATION:

1. Heat a large pan over medium flame and add sausage. Cook for about 5 minutes, breaking up meat with a spoon, until it's not pink.
2. Add the onion and sauté until softened and stir frequently. Add garlic and cook for one minute.
3. Add marinara sauce and reduce heat to medium, and simmer for 10 minutes, or until sauce starts to thicken. Stir in the pesto, salt and pepper, and adjust seasonings. Set aside.
4. In a large pot of salted boiling water, cook pasta for 10 minutes or until done *al dente*. Drain.
5. Pre-heat oven to 375 F. Oil a 9 X 13 baking dish. Spread a thin layer of sauce in the pan.
6. Combine the pasta in a large bowl with remaining sauce, 1/3 cup of Parmesan cheese, spinach, diced cheese, and mix well to combine. Spoon the mixture into the prepared pan and sprinkle remaining Parmesan cheese (2/3rds of a cup) on top.
7. Bake for about 30 minutes or until cheese is well browned.

Roasted, New Rosemary Potatoes

INGREDIENTS: 2 pounds of very small, new potatoes, either red or Yukon Gold
½ cup of olive oil
2 Tablespoons coarse sea salt
2 Tablespoons of chopped fresh rosemary

PREPARATION:

1. Preheat oven to 375 degrees.
2. Cut potatoes in half or in wedges. Toss in a bowl with all ingredients to coat them well.
3. Spread out evenly on a heavy baking sheet and bake for 20 to 30 minutes. Turn occasionally and bake until golden brown.

Roasted Pork Tenderloin
with Mushrooms and White Wine Sauce

INGREDIENTS: 1 pound of pork tenderloin
1 Tablespoon of olive oil
1 cup of sliced chanterelle or shitake mushrooms
¼ cup of white wine
¼ cup of unfiltered apple juice
2 Tablespoons of Dijon mustard
½ cup of cream

PREPARATION:

1. Brush tenderloins with olive oil and season with salt and pepper.
2. Preheat a cast iron pan or heavy pan on medium high heat and sear tenderloin until brown on all sides. Place pan in oven and roast for about 10 minutes at 375 degrees. Set pork tenderloin aside and keep warm.
3. Place the pan back on the stove top and add the sliced mushrooms and cook for 5 five minutes. Pour in the apple juice and the white wine. Blend in the mustard and simmer until liquid is reduced by half.
4. Add cream and seasons with salt and pepper to taste.
5. To serve, slice into small rounds, drizzle sauce over top and garnish with sage leaves.

Maple Spinach Salad

INGREDIENTS:
2 large bunches of fresh spinach
4 ounces of sliced mushrooms
1 hard boiled egg
8 ounces of bacon, cooked crisp
1/3 cup of maple syrup
2/3rds of a cup of aged rice wine vinegar
2 Tablespoons of roasted sesame seeds

PREPARATION:

1. Remove stems from spinach and toss with mushrooms in serving bowl.
2. Chop egg and crumble bacon. Toss with the spinach.
3. Mix maple syrup and vinegar together. Add salt and pepper.
4. Heat until warm in a sauce pan.
5. Sprinkle sesame seeds over the spinach.
6. Pour dressing over salad and toss well.

Citrus Ginger Vinaigrette

INGREDIENTS:
1 ½ cups orange juice, freshly squeezed
1 cup aged rice wine vinegar
2 cups of olive oil, extra virgin
4 Tablespoons of ginger root, finely minced
1 cup of light honey

PREPARATION:

1. Add all ingredients to blender except olive oil. Blend on high until mixture is smooth (about one minute).
2. Slowly add olive oil with blender on high until all oil is incorporated.
3. Salt and pepper to taste.
4. Use as a dressing for mixed greens, marinade for chicken or dipping sauce for asparagus. Makes 4 cups.

Balsamic Maple Vinaigrette

INGREDIENTS:
¼ cup reduced balsamic vinegar
½ cup pure maple syrup
1 Tablespoon lemon juice
1 cup extra virgin olive oil
½ Teaspoon dried basil

1 Teaspoon dry mustard
1 clove of garlic, finely minced
¼ Teaspoon of black pepper
1 Teaspoon of salt

PREPARATION: ···

1. Buy inexpensive balsamic vinegar and cook on stove until reduced by half. Store in refrigerator for other uses.
2. For this recipe, put all ingredients in blender, except olive oil and salt and pepper. Blend well and then slowly add olive oil.
3. Remove from blender and whisk in salt and pepper.
4. This keeps in refrigerator for up to two weeks.

◌℮◌

Quinoa & Veggie Souffle

INGREDIENTS: ¾ cup quinoa
1 ½ cups water
3 Tablespoons of oil, divided
2 ½ cups grated carrots
1 ½ Tablespoons dried thyme, divided
2 ½ cups grated zucchini
1 medium yellow onion, diced into ½ pieces
1 cup grated Asiago cheese
2 cups ricotta cheese
1 ½ Tablespoons sea salt
½ Teaspoon pepper
2 Tablespoons chopped fresh basil
4 eggs separated

PREPARATION: ···

1. Place quinoa in a fine sieve and rinse well.
2. In a saucepan on medium heat, stir in the quinoa and stir for about 5 minutes or until it has a nutty aroma. Add water, lower heat to simmer, cover and cook for 10 minutes, then set aside to cool.
3. In a saucepan, add one tablespoon of oil and sauté grated carrots with ½ tsp. of dried thyme. Set aside.
4. Sauté zucchini and onion separately, using same method as the carrots. Place all vegetables in a mixing bowl and add cheese and mix well.
5. Add salt and pepper and basil. Beat egg yolks and add to mixture and stir well.
6. Beat egg whites until they have stiff peaks and gently fold into the mixture.
7. Oil a 6 inch soufflé pan and pour the mixture into it. Cover and bake in preheated oven at 350 degrees to 30 minutes. Uncover and bake 30 minutes more.
8. Soufflé is done when a knife inserted into it comes out clean. Serve immediately.

Santa Barbara Couscous

INGREDIENTS, DRESSING:
½ Teaspoon cumin
½ Teaspoon cardamom
¼ Teaspoon cinnamon
¼ cup lemon juice
¼ cup orange juice
1 Teaspoon minced, fresh ginger (about a one inch piece)
1 Tablespoon of honey
½ Tablespoon of lemon zest
¼ cup of olive oil

INGREDIENTS, SALAD:
1 ½ cups of Israeli Couscous or regular, if unavailable
1 ½ cups of water
¼ Teaspoon tumeric
1 small red pepper, seeded, and finely chopped
1 small yellow pepper, seeded and finely chopped
½ small red onion, seeded and chopped
10 dried figs, finely sliced
10 dried apricots, sliced
½ cup of raisins, golden flame raisins, or others
1 cup, shelled pistachio nuts, toasted and chopped
½ cup of minced fresh cilantro
1 ½ Tablespoons grated orange zest

PREPARATION:

1. Combine all ingredients for dressing. May be made ahead and kept in refrigerator.
2. Preheat oven to 375 degrees and place couscous in baking pan. Roast for 10 minutes until couscous turns golden brown. Cool down and place in a bowl.
3. Combine water with tumeric and bring to a boil. Add couscous and bring to a boil.
4. Simmer for 10 to 15 minutes with cover on pot.
5. Set aside and leave cover on for 10 minutes.
6. Fluff couscous with fork.
7. Turn out into serving bowl and add all other ingredients.
8. Add dressing and mix well.
9. Enjoy!

Spinach, Basil, and Lemon Pesto

INGREDIENTS:
1 ½ cups fresh basil
½ cup fresh spinach
1 Tablespoon grated lemon zest
½ cup freshly grated Parmesan cheese
½ cup olive oil
½ cup freshly squeezed lemon juice (2 to 3 juicy lemons)
¼ cup walnuts, toasted
4 cloves of minced garlic
Salt and freshly ground pepper, *al gusto*

PREPARATION:

1. Use food processor and combine all ingredients and puree until smooth.
2. Keeps in refrigerator for up to one week or in freezer for up to 3 months.

Santa Barbara Summer Pesto

INGREDIENTS:
4 cups fresh basil leaves (1/4 lb. tightly packed)
1 cup of pine nuts
1 cup, freshly grated Parmesan or Romano cheese
5 cloves of garlic
3 Tablespoons lemon juice
1 cup, olive oil
1 Teaspoon of salt
1 Teaspoon of pepper

PREPARATION:

1. Toast nuts in 225 degree oven for 15 minutes, or until browned.
2. Chop garlic fine in food processor.
3. Add basil leaves, sprinkle with lemon juice, salt and pepper.
4. Add cooled pine nuts.
5. Turn on motor and add olive oil in a thin stream through the feed tube.
6. Process until mixture is smooth.
7. Remove from food processor and mix with grated cheese.

Vietnamese Favorites

I urge you to eat Vietnamese and Thai food every chance you can. They're some of the world's most highly evolved and healthy cuisines. Rich in coconut milks, fresh sea foods, fish sauce, lettuce, pork and finely sliced beef, aromatic mints, herbs, sesame, rice, spices; they're nourishing for both the body and the soul.

Hanoi Grilled Pork

(Serves 4)

INGREDIENTS:
- 1 Tablespoon of honey
- 2 Tablespoons fish sauce
- 1 large shallot
- 1 clove of minced garlic
- 2 Tablespoons palm sugar (or honey)
- 1 Teaspoon of sea salt or *Real Salt*
- 1 lb. minced boneless pork loin
- 8 oz. cooked rice noodles
- Lettuce leaves
- 4 oz. mung bean sprouts
- Handful of coriander, basil leaves, mint leaves and chives

CUCUMBER DIPPING SAUCE: Mix all ingredients in bowl:
- ½ cucumber, peeled, deseeded and grated
- Juice of two limes
- 2 Tablespoons fish sauce
- 1 small red chili, chopped very fine
- 1 large garlic clove, chopped fine
- 1 Teaspoon of honey
- Season with salt and pepper to taste

PREPARATION:

1. Mix the honey with 2/3rds of the fish sauce in a sauce pan and stir constantly. Transfer to a bowl and combine with garlic, shallot, palm sugar, remaining fish sauce and salt. Add minced pork, cover and let stand for 3 hours.
2. Shape the minced pork mixture into 20 to 24 patties about once inch in diameter and place under a pre-heated grill and cook for 3 to 4 minutes on each side until cooked through. They're also excellent to barbecue.
3. To serve, divide the rice noodles between 4 warmed bowls and add the pork, lettuce leaves, bean sprouts and herbs. Spoon dipping sauce over the mixture.

Sizzling Turmeric Catfish

In this recipe, I sometimes substitute English Sole,
Dover Sole or local Petrali Sole for the catfish.

INGREDIENTS: 1 lb. fresh, white meat fish
2 green onion stalks
1 brown onion
Marinade (see below)
Mixed greens (see below)
Dipping Sauce (see at end of Preparation)
12 Rice Paper rounds (Rice paper rounds are made from
ground, cooked rice and water. This batter is cooked over a fire,
then each round is then dried on a bamboo mat. Buy them in
Asian markets.)

PREPARATION: ....

1. PREPARE FISH MIXTURE: Cut fish into small pieces (about 1 inch by 2 inches),
and mix with green onion stalks (cut into 1 ½ inch pieces) and 1 brown onion
(thinly sliced). Let this mixture sit in Marinade Sauce.

2. PREPARE MARINADE SAUCE:
Mix well to marinate fish pieces:
2 Tablespoons of honey
2 Teaspoons of turmeric
1 Teaspoon of olive oil
½ cup freshly chopped fresh dill, and a pinch of salt.

3. PREPARE FRESH MIXED GREENS:
Wash and dry, then coarsely chop and set aside:
1 bunch of green leaf lettuce
1 large bunch of mint leaves
1 bunch of cilantro
1 thinly sliced cucumber (preferably English or hot house)
½ pound of mung bean sprouts

4. Heat wok or very large pan to highest heat. When very hot, add cooking oil. Add
fish and onion mixture.

5. Toss well and season with sea salt. Remove from heat and serve immediately.

6. Use a large bowl and fill with warm water and soak rice paper rounds. Submerge
whole rice paper round. Let soak until soft and remove from water. Then place on
cutting board or serving platter. (It takes about 2 minutes of soaking to soften them.
If serving for guests, have each diner prepare their own.)

7. Place 2 or 3 pieces of catfish and onions on center of rice paper along with assorted
fresh greens. Fold both pieces of rice paper and roll up like a burrito.

Dip in Dipping sauce — one dip for each bite. Enjoy!

8. **VIETNAMESE DIPPING SAUCE:**

Mix all ingredients well:

½ cup of warmed honey
½ cup of water
¼ cup of fish sauce
¼ cup of aged rice wine vinegar
2 Tablespoons of finely minced garlic
2 teaspoons of chili paste
2 finely chopped Thai chilies (optional)

Glazed Tofu

This is good served on a plate of fresh spinach and with a side of hot rice.

INGREDIENTS: 1 carton of firm tofu
2 or 3 cloves of garlic, coarsely chopped
2 Tablespoons of fresh lime or lemon juice
¼ cup good soy sauce
¼ cup sweet soy sauce (Indonesian style is best)
2 Teaspoons of sesame oil
3 Tablespoons of chopped cilantro
Salt and pepper
2 Tablespoons of coconut or peanut oil for frying

PREPARATION:

1. Drain tofu well.
2. Place tofu on cutting block and carefully slice in half horizontally. Square up stack and cut tofu in X pattern, making 4 triangles. Cut again in + pattern to make a total of 16 small triangles.
3. Combine all ingredients.
4. Heat up cooking oil, until very hot and add tofu.
5. Cook over medium high heat without disturbing until golden crispy, about 7 minutes. Pour in the marinade and shuffle pan back and forth to coat tofu. Use cornstarch and water if needed to thicken.
6. Reduce heat to medium and cook until sauce is syrupy. Serve immediately.

Cilantro Crab Cakes

INGREDIENTS: 1 lb. can of good crab meat or use freshly picked crab meat
2 Tablespoons of diced shallots
1 cup of bread crumbs or Panko crumbs

2 Tablespoons of finely chopped cilantro
2 eggs, slightly beaten
1 Teaspoon of Worchester sauce
1 Teaspoon of soy sauce
A few drops of Tabasco sauce
Coconut oil for frying

PREPARATION: ··

1. Combine shallot, crabmeat, cilantro and breadcrumbs in a bowl and mix well.
2. Mix eggs, soy sauce, Worcestershire sauce, and Tabasco well in a small bowl.
3. Stir egg mixture into crabmeat mixture and blend until all crabmeat lumps are broken up.
4. Set skillet on medium high with 2 Tablespoons of coconut oil and cook cakes until golden brown on both sides.

Serve with dipping sauce. Enjoy!

DIPPING SAUCE: Mix well:
¼ cup of peanut oil
½ cup of lime juice
2 Tablespoons of chopped lemon grass
3 teaspoons of soy sauce
2 Tablespoons of honey, 1 drop of Tabasco sauce.

Vietnamese Peanut Sauce

INGREDIENTS: 2 Tablespoons of warm coconut or peanut oil
12 shallots, finely chopped
1 Teaspoon of cayenne
1 Teaspoon of shrimp paste (Leave out if you don't have it, or use fish sauce.)
4 Tablespoons of finely chopped lemon grass
4 Tablespoons of peanut butter
8 oz. of canned or frozen coconut milk
2 Tablespoons of chopped fresh cilantro

PREPARATION: ··

1. Heat oil and sauté shallots, shrimp paste, cayenne and lemon grass until fragrant, about 5 minutes.
2. Add coconut milk and peanut butter and cook about 10 to 15 minutes.
3. Stir constantly. Remove from heat and mix in cilantro.

Diet Style-Bananas in Coconut Milk

INGREDIENTS:
3 cans of coconut milk (or frozen, if you can find it)
4 large, ripe bananas
2/3 cup of honey
1 Tablespoon vanilla
¼ cup small tapioca pearls
2/3 cup of water
Toasted sesame seeds
¼ teaspoon of salt

PREPARATION:

1. Soak tapioca pearls in warm water for 20 minutes. Drain and set aside.
2. Combine water, coconut milk, honey, salt and vanilla in sauce pan at high heat. Don't let it boil over.
3. Reduce heat to medium low.
4. Add tapioca and bananas to the mixture.
5. Serve in individual bowls and sprinkle sesame seeds on top.

Thai Foods

Chicken with Vegetables

INGREDIENTS:
- 2 Tablespoons of coconut oil
- 2 cloves of minced garlic
- 1 cup, thinly sliced chicken breast
- ¼ cup of sliced onions
- ½ cup of sliced carrots
- 1 cup of sliced cabbage
- 1 cup of broccoli flowerets
- ½ cup sliced cauliflower
- ½ cup each of sliced red and green peppers
- ¼ cup of snow peas
- ¼ cup of sliced mushrooms
- ¼ cup of bean sprouts

SAUCE:
- 1 Tablespoon of fish sauce
- 1 Tablespoon of oyster sauce
- 1 Tablespoon of honey

PREPARATION:

1. Heat oil in large sautéing pan and add garlic. Stir for a moment, then add chicken pieces. Stir well and cook chicken until nearly done.
2. Add vegetables and mixed sauce ingredients and stir fry until vegetables are crisp and tender.
3. Serve hot with brown rice.

Pineapple Curry with Shrimp

INGREDIENTS:
- 14 ounces of coconut milk (Use frozen coconut from the Philippines if you can find it in your local market.)
- 1 cup of crushed, canned pineapple (use fresh if you can)
- ¼ cup of fish sauce
- 1 ½ Tablespoons of honey
- 2 Tablespoons of lemon juice
- ½ pound of shrimp, shelled and deveined
- Garnish with thin strips of lime leaves or lime peel

PREPARATION:

1. Combine all ingredients except shrimp and bring to a boil.
2. Add shrimp and cook until done.

Beef Salad

INGREDIENTS:	½ lb. of New York Steak
	1 Tablespoon of fish sauce
	Head of leafy, green lettuce
	½ tomato, sliced into thin slices
	½ cup cucumber slices
	¼ cup sliced red and green bell peppers
	¼ cup sliced onions
	½ cup sliced mushrooms
	1 green onion, cut into one inch pieces
DRESSING:	3 Tablespoons of fish sauce
	3 Tablespoons of lime juice
	1 Tablespoon of honey
	3 cloves of garlic, minced Cilantro (for garnish)
	2 Tablespoons roasted peanuts, chopped coarsely
	2 Thai chili peppers, optional

PREPARATION:

1. Marinate steak with fish sauce for about 5 minutes.
2. Grill steak until medium rare, or how you like it, slice and set aside.
3. Line a large platter with green leaf lettuce leaves. Arrange all ingredients on top of lettuce and pour dressing over vegetables and beef.
4. Garnish with chopped cilantro and chopped peanuts.

Baked Rice in Pineapple with Cashew Nuts

INGREDIENTS:	1 whole fresh pineapple (cut in half lengthwise)
	2 Tablespoons of oil
	½ lb. of diced chicken
	1/3 cup of coconut milk
	¼ Teaspoon of white pepper
	½ cup toasted cashew nuts
	½ cup crushed pineapple
	¼ cup of golden raisins
	2 Tablespoons of chopped cilantro
	3 Cups of cooked brown basmati rice sauce:
	¼ cup fish sauce
	1 Tablespoon of sweet chili sauce
	¼ cup of honey

PREPARATION: ··

1. Cut pineapple in half, lengthwise, and remove fruit. Dice pineapple and scrape out shell, so it can be used as a serving dish.
2. Heat frying pan and add oil. Cook chicken until its 2/3rds done. Add all seasonings and cook until mixture foams.
3. Add cashews, pineapple, raisins, chopped cilantro, and rice. Turn off heat and mix well.
4. Put rice into pineapple and bake in 350 degree oven for 20 minutes or until well heated.

Thai Style, Kabocha Squash Desert

INGREDIENTS: ½ large Kabocha squash
14 oz. can of coconut milk (use frozen if you can)
¼ can of coconut sugar (substitute honey)

PREPARATION: ··

1. Peel squash and slice into one inch pieces that are ¼ thick.
2. Bring coconut milk to a boil and add coconut sugar. Stir and bring to a boil again.
3. Add sliced squash and simmer until squash is done, about 15
4. minutes.

Chinese Recipes

These are my old time, traditional Chinese recipes I used before I discovered Vietnamese and Thai foods. They're good recipes for light and healthy foods that are easy to prepare.

Sweet and Sour Bean Sprouts

INGREDIENTS: 1 pound of fresh mung bean sprouts
½ cup shredded green pepper, cut in very thin slices

SEASONINGS: ½ Teaspoon of Real Salt or Sea Salt
2 Tablespoons of honey
2 Tablespoons of rice wine vinegar
3 Tablespoons of peanut oil

PREPARATION: ··

1. Rinse bean sprouts well and dry. Mix all seasonings
2. Heat oil and add veggies when hot. Add all seasonings and
3. stir fry until crisp and tender.
4. Remove and serve hot or cold.

c

Micro-Wave-Chinese, Fast-Food Style Trout or Dover Sole Fillets

INGREDIENTS: 1 lb. of fish fillet
3 stalks of green onion
4 slices of fresh ginger
2 slices of bacon (or 2 Tablespoons of sesame oil)
1 Tablespoon of corn starch
1 Tablespoon of peanut oil

SEASONINGS: 2 Tablespoons of sherry
1 Teaspoon of salt
1 Tablespoon of soy sauce
2 Teaspoons of honey
Dash of pepper

PREPARATION: ··

1. Marinate fish fillet with seasonings for at least 2 hours.
2. Shred green onion and ginger.
3. Cut bacon into ½ pieces and cook on full power in microwave for 30 seconds. Stir and cook for another 60 to 90 seconds. Cover with paper plate while cooking.
4. Divide fish onto two plates and use flour sifter to gently sprinkle cornstarch on both sides of fillet.
5. Put ginger and green onion on top of fillet.
6. Pour bacon and bacon grease on fish. Sprinkle cooking oil on fish.
7. Cover fish with paper plate and microwave on full power for 3 minutes for each plate.

Sweet Treats

Banana Macadamia Bread

This recipe makes two 8 ½ inch loaves.
It's great topped with cream fraiche or jam.

INGREDIENTS: 16 ounces, raw unsalted macadamia nuts
¾ cup of honey
4 large, fresh eggs
4 very ripe bananas, mashed
4 tablespoons of melted butter
1 teaspoon vanilla extract
1 teaspoon baking soda

PREPARATION:

1.   Preheat oven to 300 F. Grease two 1.5 quart (8 ½ X 4 ½ X 2 ½) loaf pans and line them with parchment paper.
2.   Place all ingredients in food processor and blend until smooth. Pour batter into prepared loaf pans and bake for 55 to 60 minutes.
3.   Turn off the oven and leave loaves in until oven cools down. Remove from pans and serve. Or wrap in plastic wrap and store in refrigerator for up to 4 days.

The World's Best Cherry Pie

In making this recipe, use the best quality butter you can afford. I prefer Double Devon Cream butter and Kerrygold butters available from Trader Joe's. When you first taste them, you realize this is what butter coming from cows raised in lush green pastures tastes like. Of course, down here on blue earth, in America, fresh, local and seasonal is best, so always buy locally produced butter if it's available.)

INGREDIENTS FOR TWO PIES.... PIE FILLING:

10 cups of fresh, sour cherries
2 ½ cups of sugar
Pie crust (to make 2 pie tops and bottom crusts; 9 inch size in a deep Pyrex dish):
1 ½ cups of King Arthur bleached all purpose flour
1 ½ cups of King Arthur white whole wheat flour

2 Tsp. of *Real Salt*
1 cup of butter
A little less than 2/3 cup of water

PREPARATION: ··

1. Cut butter into small pieces and add slowly to well sifted flour and salt mixture.
2. Cut butter in with dough mixer tool or use fork.
3. Gradually add water, and mix until just barely mixed.
4. Work dough as little as possible to blend it. Use as little water as possible.
5. Add carefully, bit by bit, to make sure you don't get it too wet. Roll into ball and place in refrigerator when mix sticks together well.

PIE-MIX: ··

1. Pit all cherries. That didn't take too long, did it? Use Austrian Pie-Cherry Pitter next time...
2. Drain juice from 10 cups of cherries and save juice and drink it. It's good for you!
3. Mix 2 ½ cups of sugar with 8 Tablespoons of Pie-Filling Enhancer, (made primarily from corn starch and available from King Arthur Flour Company. Use corn starch, if you don't have pie filling enhancer.) Blend well.
4. Add cherries into a large bowl and coat well with sugar and thickener. Sprinkle the sugar mix onto them 1 or 2 cups at a time until they're well-coated. Blend carefully.

PREPARATION: ··

1. Spray pie pan with olive oil spray. Roll out pie dough on floured cloth and drape inside of pie pan and trim edges. Pierce dough in 2 or 3 places lightly with fork in bottom of pan.
2. Carefully spoon cherry, sugar and thickener mixture into pie.
3. Use lattice pie-top cutter (available from King Arthur Flour Co.) and cut out pie dough top and drape on pie. Use water to seal edges. Crimp edges well.
4. Cook pies at 350 degrees until done, about 70 minutes. Cover pies with aluminum foil while baking except for the last 20 minutes.

cℓ⌒

High-Tech, Santa Barbara Rich Kid Version of The World's Best Cherry Pie

Follow all the same instructions for recipe above, except:

1. Cut pie dough recipe in half to make one pie.
2. Use 4 lb bag of frozen berries from Costco (raspberries, blueberries and marionberry mix)
3. Drain bag well—this makes 4 to 5 cups of berries.
4. Use ¾ cup of sugar and 4 tablespoons of pie enhancer.

cℓ⌒

Lemon Coconut Macaroons

INGREDIENTS: Egg whites from 7 large eggs
2 ½ teaspoons vanilla extract
1/8 teaspoon *Real Salt* or finely ground sea salt (use mortar and pestle)
1 ½ Tablespoons grated lemon zest
¾ cup of Santa Barbara honey, if you can get it
3 cups shredded, unsweetened coconut

PREPARATION:

1. Preheat oven to 250 F. Line two cookie sheets with parchment paper.
2. Use electric mixer and beat egg whites with salt on high speed until stiff peaks form. Gently fold in all other ingredients until well mixed.
3. Drop tablespoonfuls of batter with one inch spacing on cookie sheets. Bake for one hour and let cool to make chewy cookies. Store in airtight jar in refrigerator.

Orange-Vanilla-Honey Smoothie

INGREDIENTS: 2 cups freshly squeezed orange juice
1 cup of plain, full fat yoghurt
¼ cup of honey (slightly warmed)
2 cups of ice cubes
1 Tablespoon of pure vanilla extract
1 orange, cut into slices for garnish

PREPARATION:

1. Combine all ingredients in a blender, until ice cubes turn into slush.
2. Pour into glasses and garnish with orange slices.

Mary's Minnesota Summer Sherbet

INGREDIENTS: 2 bananas
2 oranges
2 lemons
1 ½ cups of honey
2 beaten eggs
1 cup of water
1 cup of whole raw milk

PREPARATION: ··

1.   Juice lemons, oranges, and mash bananas.
2.   Mix in eggs, honey, water and milk and mix well.
3.   Put in shallow tray to freeze.
4.   After it starts to freeze a little bit, stir with a fork again. Thishelps to break up crystals.
5.   Freeze solid.
6.   This is a good mix to use in Popsicle molds.

Indian Pudding

Always a holiday favorite — the traditional New England Dish. Make it with whole certified raw milk and organic cornmeal for a true taste treat. Serve with cream fraiche or the very finest vanilla ice cream.

INGREDIENTS: ¼ cup cornmeal
3 cups of milk
1 egg
¼ cup of honey
½ cup of molasses
1 Tablespoon of butter
1 Teaspoon of cinnamon
½ Teaspoon of ginger

PREPARATION: ··

1.   Mix ¼ cup of cornmeal into one cup of cold salted water.
2.   Stir in two cups of scalded milk and bring to a boil.
3.   Boil for 10 minutes.
4.   Blend in one well beaten egg, honey, molasses, and spices.
5.   Butter casserole dish and bake for 30 minutes at 300 degrees.
6.   Remove from oven and stir in 1 cup of cold milk. Mix well.
7.   Bake two more hours at 300 degrees.

Cashew Cookies

Earlier in the book, I said I would give some recipes for those afflicted with Crohn's disease. The Cashew Cookies and the following Crohnie Brownies are healthy fare for those afflicted with this disease. For those with IBS, celiac disease, or Crohn's Disease — diseases for which modern medicine has little help— — changing your diet works wonders. An excellent reference book is the new book, Eat Well–Live Well, by Montecito cooking savant, Kendall Conrad. It's a "must have" for anyone with eating disorders. It also names Santa Barbara doctors who have developed dietary regimens for those afflicted with these diseases.

INGREDIENTS:
1 cup raw almonds
½ cup extra virgin coconut oil
1 cup fresh cashew butter (It's best to grind all nuts at the store where you buy them to assure freshness)
½ cup local honey
¼ Teaspoon salt
2 eggs
¼ Teaspoon baking soda
1 Teaspoon vanilla

PREPARATION:
1. Pour almonds into blender and grind to a flour.
2. Mix with the rest of the ingredients, put in a large bowl, cover and refrigerate.
3. When it's hardened, it can be scooped out and baked on a large cookie sheet that's been sprayed with olive oil.
4. Bake until golden, about 8 minutes.

Crohnie Brownies

INGREDIENTS:
¾ cup of raw almonds
6 ounces of virgin coconut oil (The whiter the better---when it comes to coconut oil)
1 cup Santa Barbara honey (Buy it at the Farmer's Market if you live in Santa Barbara)
3 eggs
½ cup, well packed, unsweetened natural cocoa powder
1 Teaspoon of vanilla
½ Teaspoon of salt
½ cup of chopped walnuts

¾ Teaspoon of baking soda

PREPARATION: ···

1. Preheat oven to 350 degrees.
2. Pour almonds in blender and grind to a flour.
3. Mix well with rest of ingredients.
4. Spray a 9 X 9 baking pan with oil and bake for 35 to 40 minutes.

Teff Pudding

Teff is native to the highlands of Ethiopia and is made into the tangy, sourdough bread known as injera. Teff is the world's smallest grain and is also the most nutritious grain in the world. It's also extremely high in iron — a good grain for your health!

INGREDIENTS: 2 cups of water
½ cup of teff grain
2 large ripe bananas
2 Tablespoons maple syrup, honey, agave syrup or brown rice syrup
2 Teaspoons of vanilla
3 Tablespoons of cocoa powder

PREPARATION: ···

1. In a medium size pot, bring the water and the Teff to a boil. Cover and simmer over low heat until water is absorbed. (15 to 20 minutes)
2. Stir occasionally. Let cool and mix in a blender with all other ingredients.
3. Add additional water if needed.
4. Pour into serving bowls and chill.

Healthy Breakfasts

Uncle Nick's Oat and Whole Wheat Waffles

INGREDIENTS:
3 cups of oats
¾ cup whole wheat flour
4 cups of buttermilk or raw milk
2 large eggs or 3 small ones
1 ½ Teaspoon of baking powder
½ Teaspoon of Real Salt
1 Teaspoon of vanilla
Huckleberries or blueberries for topping

PREPARATION:

1. Put oats in a large mixing bowl and add milk and vanilla. and let sit for at least half an hour, preferably overnight.
2. Measure whole wheat flour into smaller bowl and mix well with salt and baking powder.
3. Break eggs into large bowl and remove yolks and mix them.
4. Whip egg whites, add vanilla, and beat until peaks are standing tall and very stiff.
5. Add beaten egg yolks to milk mixture. Mix well. Then slowly add whole wheat mixture.
6. Gently fold in beaten egg whites.
7. Heat waffle iron and brush or spray with oil between waffles.
8. Make the first waffle a small one and throw it away.
9. Use pure butter and maple syrup and add huckleberries and blueberries to your taste.

Seafood and Wild Game Recipes

Hawaiian Style, Macadamia Nut Crusted Mahi-Mahi with Chile Flavored Coconut Butter Sauce

INGREDIENTS:
- 2 Mahi-Mahi fillets, 6 oz. each
- 1 cup Panko bread crumbs
- 1/8 cup chopped macadamia nuts
- 2 Teaspoons of grated ginger
- Salt and pepper to taste
- Equal parts of coconut oil and butter for cooking

PREPARATION:

1. Blend crumbs, nuts, and ginger in food processor and chop until fine.
2. Season fillets with salt and pepper.
3. Coat fillets with breadcrumb mixture.
4. Sauté fish in coconut oil and butter until golden brown and just barely cooked through.

SAUCE:
- ½ cup of white wine
- ¾ cup of coconut crème (usually canned)
- ½ cup chicken broth
- 1 Tablespoon finely chopped shallots
- ½ Teaspoon of finely chopped ginger
- ½ Teaspoon sweet Thai or Indonesian chili sauce
- 1 Tablespoon chopped basil
- 2 Tablespoons of soft butter

PREPARATION:

1. In small sauce pan combine first 5 ingredients and simmer until sauce is reduced by about half.
2. Add chili sauce and basil and slowly whisk in butter until it's incorporated into the sauce.
3. Place Mahi-Mahi fillets on serving platter and drizzle with sauce.

Tempura Fried Trout Eggs

After reading about the travels of nutritional pioneer Weston Price in the 1920s and 1930s, I decided I'd share this recipe with you. Dr. Price discovered that primitive cultures enjoying incredibly good health valued fish eggs and sea food very highly. Interesting, isn't it? What we "civilized" folks throw away is exactly what so-called primitive peoples value most.

Last fall when I went trout fishing, I figured out a recipe for eating fish eggs. What I did was batter them up with tempura and use a dipping sauce. Why not let Mother Nature provide you with the world's finest vitamins and minerals?

INGREDIENTS:	Freshly caught trout or salmon eggs
	Coconut oil for frying, or use Mary's Blend of 1/3rd coconut oil, 1/3 sesame oil and 1/3 olive oil.
TEMPURA BATTER:	1 egg white
	2 Tablespoons cornstarch
	½ Teaspoon of baking powder
	2 Tablespoons of water
	1 Tablespoon of coconut oil

PREPARATION:

1. Beat egg white stiffly
2. Add corn starch and remaining ingredients.
3. Cut fish eggs in 1 inch pieces.
4. Batter fish eggs well and fry in hot oil at 350 to 375 degrees.

Steamed Mussels with Tomatoes (Basque Style)

INGREDIENTS:	8 Tablespoons (one stick of unsalted butter)
	4 cups of chopped tomatoes
	3 garlic cloves, minced
	1 Teaspoon of *Real Salt*, or sea salt
	1/3 loaf of crusty, day old bread
	1 cup of dry white wine
	4 lbs of fresh mussels, cleaned and debearded
	3 Tablespoons, chopped, fresh parsley
	3 Tablespoons, finely chopped chives

PREPARATION: ··

1. Melt butter in a large saucepan over medium-high heat.
2. Add garlic and sauté for one minute, and then add tomatoes and sauté for 4 or 5 more minutes.
3. Add salt and pepper to taste, wine and bread cubes, and let simmer for 5 or 6 minutes.
4. Add the mussels, cover and simmer until they open in about 6 or 8 minutes. Stir mussels gently every few minutes to make sure they cook evenly. Discard any that don't open.
5. Serve in shallow bowls and garnish with chives and parsley.

Glory Days Scallop Soup

INGREDIENTS: ½ pound of small scallops or ½ pound of chopped large ones, if possible from the Santa Barbara Channel Islands.
6 cups of homemade chicken broth
6 thin slices of fresh ginger
2 green onions
1 sweet red pepper
12 springs of fresh cilantro
2 eggs from lively free range chickens
1 Tablespoon of dry sherry
2 Teaspoons of sesame oil
¼ Teaspoon of freshly ground white pepper
½ to one Teaspoon of salt

PREPARATION: ··

1. Shred the green onions, stem and seed the peppers and chop them.
2. Cook broth with ginger slices for 15 minutes and discard ginger.
3. Bring broth to a low boil and add scallops.
4. Beat eggs and mix well. Add 2 or 3 Tablespoons of warm broth to eggs to warm them. Stir broth.
5. When it begins to boil again, add eggs in thin stream and stir where eggs hit hot liquid.
6. Stir in sherry, lemon juice, sesame oil, white pepper, and salt to taste.
7. Stir in green onions, red pepper, chopped cilantro, and serve at once.

Ultimate Abalone

We have to wait a few more years until the protection of the abalones at the Channel Islands gathers some critical mass. Hopefully, in 2008, a sport diving abalone season will open up again. In this recipe, red abalone will do — pink abalone is better, and deepwater white abalone is the best of them all. Sadly, white abalones are now on the endangered species list.

INGREDIENTS: Abalone, trimmed down to white meat only, sliced very thinly, beaten and pounded with a mallet. (Use a plastic one with a weighted, textured head.)
Whole wheat pastry flour or white whole wheat
Beaten eggs
Panko breadcrumbs and seasoned breadcrumbs, salt and pepper blended together.
Peanut oil for frying

PREPARATION:

1. Roll abalone in flour.
2. Dip abalone in beaten egg.
3. Roll in bread crumb mixture.
4. Cook in peanut oil or grape seed oil heated enough to almost smoke.
5. Cook quickly, 5 to 10 seconds on each side—as little as you need to cook them.
6. Store in warmed oven and keep warm until finished.

Nutritious Quick Meals for Families

My intention in writing these recipes is to give people healthy foods cooked from natural ingredients. I certainly realize that people are on the go more than ever, so the following recipes use canned foods and are good choices for those who don't have the time to cook everything from scratch.

Fish In The Tomato Patch Stew

INGREDIENTS:
- 1 pound of firm fish, cut into 2 to 3 inch chunks
- 3 ½ ounces sun dried tomatoes
- 2 Tablespoons olive oil
- 1 large yellow onion, chopped
- 1 green bell pepper, chopped
- 2-8 ounce bottles clam juice
- 2-14 ounce cans diced tomatoes (no salt added)
- 1 cup of red wine (or substitute broth or tomato juice)
- 4 garlic cloves, minced
- 4 Tablespoons of fresh herbs (thyme, rosemary or basil) or
- 2 Tablespoons dried
- ½ cup of kalamata olives, sliced
- 15 ounce can of navy beans, drained
- 2 Tablespoons fennel seeds, lightly crushed
- Salt and pepper, to taste
- ½ cup grated Parmesan cheese

PREPARATION:

1. Simmer sun dried tomatoes in pan with 1 ½ cups of water until soft. Discard water.
2. In a large pot, sauté onion and green peppers until soft.
3. Use blender to blend sun dried tomatoes and one bottle of clam juice. Add to pot.
4. Stir in remaining clam juice, diced tomatoes, wine, garlic, herbs, bay leaves and olives.
5. Simmer twenty minutes. Add beans, fish, fennel seeds, salt and pepper. Simmer until fish is done, about 10 minutes.
6. Remove bay leaves. Ladle into bowls and sprinkle with cheese.

Baked Mustard Chicken

INGREDIENTS: ¾ cup dry, seasoned bread crumbs
¾ cup Panko bread crumbs
3 Tablespoons chopped parsley
1 Tablespoon minced garlic
1 ½ Teaspoons chopped tarragon
8 chicken legs, thigh and drumstick attached
6 Tablespoons of Dijon mustard
Salt and pepper to taste

PREPARATION:

1. Preheat oven to 350 degrees.
2. Combine all ingredients except mustard in wide, shallow bowl and mix well.
3. Use kitchen shear and trim excess skin from thigh end of chicken. Use pastry brush and lightly paint mustard on chicken legs, then season with salt and pepper.
4. Coat legs with breadcrumb mixture and place in single layer in large roasting pan.
5. Bake for 50 to 55 minutes or until completely cooked.

Honey Curry Glazed Chicken

Kids love it!

INGREDIENTS: 12 chicken drumsticks
2 Tablespoons Dijon mustard
¼ cup lemon juice
¼ cup natural honey
¼ Teaspoon mild curry powder
½ Teaspoon of salt

PREPARATION:

1. Preheat the oven to 375 degrees.
2. In a large bowl, combine mustard, lemon juice, honey, curry powder, and salt. Add the chicken and stir to coat. (This can be done ahead of time and you can refrigerate overnight.)
3. Bake for one hour. Turn once and baste occasionally. Cook until the chicken almost falls off the bone and sauce has thickened.

Brown Rice Confetti

You can use brown rice that's been previously frozen to make a quick, nutritious, inexpensive meal. Brown rice is far more nutritious than white rice but takes much longer to cook. Cook rice with chicken or vegetable stock, or water saved from steaming vegetables for additional nutritional boost. Freeze brown rice in 2 cup portions so you can make a recipe like this quickly when you don't have much time. For additional nutrition, add chopped mung bean or lentil sprouts, and stir in just before serving.

INGREDIENTS:
2 Teaspoons of coconut oil
1 large onion, chopped (about one cup)
½ cup of toasted pine nuts or almonds, walnuts or pistachio nuts
2 Teaspoons of minced garlic
½ cup of frozen corn kernels
½ cup of frozen peas
2 cups of thawed out brown rice (cooked)

PREPARATION:

1. Heat the oil and sauté the onion and the garlic.
2. Add the nuts when they're about halfway done.
3. Add the corn and the peas and cook for about one minute.
4. Warm the rice in a microwave or in the oven and add to the mixture and stir well.

Chapter End Notes

The following endnotes are intended as references
for information presented in each chapter.

CHAPTER ONE—How To Be a Healthy Human Being

For how much healthier Americans were in the 1920s, see: Fallon, Sally and Enig, Mary

G, "Americans Now and Then." *Price Pottenger Nutrition Foundation Health Journal*, 1996; also posted at www.westonprice.org

Vietnam, A Complete Photographic History, Michael Maclear. Black Dog & Leventhal Press, 2003. I quote from page 456: "After the total leveling of one town, Ben Tre, an American officer stated, "We had to destroy it to save it.'"

Bourne, GH, "The Effect of Vitamin C on the Healing of Wounds," *Proceedings of the Nutrition Society,* 1946

Pinnell, SR, "Regulation of Collagen Synthesis." *Journal of Investigative Dermatology,* 1982

Fighting the Food Giants, Paul Stitt. Natural Press, 1980

How to Live Longer and Feel Better, Linus Pauling. W.H. Freeman & Co, 1986

The Heart Revolution: The Extraordinary Discovery That Finally Laid the Cholesterol Myth to Rest, Kilmer McCully, M.D. First Harper-Perennial Edition, 2000

Study published in 1996 American Oil Chemists Society Proceedings showed that for Calcium to be effectively utilized in our bones, at least 50% of dietary fats consumed should be saturated fats.

Fallon, Sally and Mary G. Enig, PhD, "Guts and Grease: The Diet of Native Americans." Posted in the Archives online at www.westonprice.org

See Tara Parker-Pope in Health Journal in *Wall St. Journal*, Wednesday, August 9th, 2006, for how saturated fats eaten with vegetables increase absorption of vitamins and minerals.

Enzyme Nutrition—The Food Enzyme Concept, Dr. Edward Howell. Avery Publishing, 1985

Naurath HJ, Joosten E, Riezler R. "Effects of vitamin B12, folate, and

Vitamin B6 supplements in elderly people with normal serum vitamin concentrations." *The Lancet*, 1995

Rath M, Pauling L, "Solution to the puzzle of human cardiovascular disease: Its primary cause is ascorbate deficiency, leading to the deposition of lipoprotein (a) and fibrinogen/fibrin in the vascular wall." *Journal of Ortho Medicine*, 1991

Rhoads GG, Dahlen G, Berg K, Morton NE, Dannenberg AL, "Lp (a) Lipoprotein as a risk factor for myocardial infarction." *Journal of the American Medical Association*, 1986

Iseri LT, "Magnesium and cardiac arrhythmias." *Magnesium*, 1986

Iseri LT, French JH, "Magnesium: Nature's physiologic calcium blocker." *American Heart Journal*, 1984.

Teo KK, Salim Y, "Role of magnesium in reducing mortality in acute myocardial infarction: A review of the evidence." *Drugs*, 1993

Turlapaty P, Altura BM, "Magnesium deficiency produces spasms of coronary arteries:

Relationship to etiology of sudden death ischemic heart disease." *Science*, 1980

Widman L, et.al, "The dose dependent reduction in blood pressure through administration of magnesium. A double blind placebo-controlled cross over study." *American Journal of Hypertension*, 1993

CHAPTER TWO—Eat Your Cholesterol, It's Good for You!

Stop Worrying About Cholesterol—Better Ways to Avoid a Heart Attack and Get

Healthy, by Richard E. Tapert, D.O. Infinity Publishing Co., 2005

Why Animals Don't Get Heart Attacks---But People Do by Mathias Rath, M.D. MR Publishing Inc., 2003

Keys A. "Atherosclerosis: A problem in newer public health." *Journal of Mt. Sinai Hospital*, 1953

The Cholesterol Myths—Exposing the Fallacy that Saturated Fat and Cholesterol Cause Heart Disease, Uffe Ravnskov, MD, PhD. New Trends Publishing, 2000

Mann, GV, "Diet-Heart: End of an Era." *New England Journal of Medicine*, 1977

Shaper, AG, "Cardiovascular Studies in the Samburu tribe of northern Kenya." *American Heart Journal*, 1962. Camel Herdsman in Somalia living almost entirely on camel's milk also have very low cholesterol values, as shown in: Lapiccirella V, et al, *Bulletin of the World Health Organization*, 1962.

Castelli WP, Anderson KM, and Levy D, "Cholesterol and mortality: Thirty years of follow-up from the Framingham study." *Journal of the American Medical Society*, April 24, 1987

Woodhams, David J, "Nutritional deficiencies in soy protein-based infant formulas." Paper presented to the New Zealand Ministry of Health, March 5, 1995.

Know Your Fats: The Complete Primer for Understanding the Nutrition of Fats, Oils and Cholesterol, Mary G. Enig. Bethesda Press, 2000

Smart Fats: How Dietary Fats and Oils Affect Mental, Physical and Emotional Intelligence, Michael Schmidt. Frog Ltd. Berkeley, CA., 1997

Enig, Mary G, PhD, "Health and Nutritional Benefits from Coconut Oil: An Important Functional Food for the 21st Century." Presented at the AVOC Lauric Oils Symposium, Ho Chi Minh City, Vietnam, April 25, 1996.

Kabara, JJ, "Health Oils from the Tree of Life" (Nutritional and Health Aspects of Coconut Oil) *Indian Coconut Journal*, 2000

Enos WE, Holmes RH, and Beyer J, "Coronary Disease among United States soldiers killed in action in Korea." *JAMA*,1953.

Chinese Red Yeast Rice, Rita Elkins, M.H. Woodland Publishing, Utah, 1998

"Statin Drugs—A Critical Review of the Risk/Benefit Clinical Research," Joel Kaufman, Ph.D. www.drugintel.com

The Cholesterol Controversy, Edward Pinkney, MD. Daimon Verlag, 1978 1973

The Heart Revolution—The Extraordinary Discovery that Finally Laid the Cholesterol Myth to Rest, Kilmer S. McCully, MD. First Harper-Perennial Edition, 2000

Folkers K, et al, "Lovastin decreases coenzyme Q-10 levels in humans." *Proceedings of the National Academy of Sciences,* 1990

Brown, MS, "Coenzyme Q.sub.10 with HMG-CoA reductase inhibitors," United States Patent 4,933,165, Assigned Merck & Co., 1990

Tolbert, JA, "Coenzyme A.sub.10 with HMG-CoA reductase inhibitors," United States Patent 4,929 Assigned Merck & Co. Rathway, N.J.

1990

Max Planck's quote is taken from "Wissenschaftliche Selbstbiographie. Mit einem

Bildnis und der von Max von Laue gehaltenen Traueransprache." Leipzig, 1948. Scientific Autobiography and Other Papers, trans. F. Gaynor. New York, 1949 (as cited in T.S Kuhn, The Structure of Scientific Revolution.

CHAPTER 3 – The Homocysteine Revolution

His Excellency, George Washington by Joseph T. Ellis. Alfred A. Knopf, 2004

Current Biography Yearbook, published by The HW Wilson Company New York, 2007

The Heart Revolution—The Extraordinary Discovery that Finally Laid the Cholesterol Myth to Rest, Kilmer S. McCully, MD. First Harper-Perennial Edition, 2000

Rimm EB, et al, "Folate and vitamin B6 from diet and supplements in relation to risk of coronary heart disease among women." *Journal of the American Medical Association*, 1998

Selhub J, et al, "Vitamin status and intake as primary determinants of homocysteinemia in an elderly population." *Journal of the American Medical Association* 1993

Schroeder, HA, "Losses of vitamins and trace minerals resulting from processing and preservation of foods." *American Journal of Clinical Nutrition* 1971

Alfthan GA, et al, "Plasma homocysteine and cardiovascular disease mortality." *Lancet,* 1997

Havlik RJ and Feinleib, M, eds. *Proceedings for the Conference on Decline in Coronary Heart Disease Mortality.* Bethesda: NIH Publication No. 79-1610, 1979

The China Study: The Most Comprehensive Study of Nutrition Ever Conducted and the Startling Implications for Diet, Weight Loss and Long-Term Health, T. Colin Campbell and Thomas M. Campbell. Benbella Books, 2005

Mao, The Unknown Story, Jung Chang and Jan Holliday. Alfred A. Knopf, 2005

Freakonomics: A Rogue Economist Explores the Hidden Side of Everything, Steven D. Levitt and Stephen J. Dubner. William

Morrow, 2005

The Second Billion, Penny Kane. Penguin, 1987

Red and Expert, Ruth Gamberg. Schocken, 1977

Robert Bazell, Chief Science and Health Correspondent, "Is this Celebrity Doctor's Pitch

Right for You?" *NBC News,* Dec. 5, 2005

Why We Get Sick-The New Science of Darwinian Medicine, Randolph M. Nesse, MD and

George C. Williams, PhD, Vintage Books, 1996

Robert J. Davis, "Not all Forms of Vitamin E Should be Vilified." *Wall St. Journal,*

Nov. 23, 2004

Finnish-Harvard study results are reported in Knekt P, et al, "Antioxidant vitamins and

coronary heart disease risk: a pooled analysis of 9 cohorts. *American Journal of Clinical Nutrition*, December 2004

According to the World Health Organization, China now rates last among developing countries in terms of equal access to medical care. See Elisabeth Rosenthal, "Without 'Barefoot Doctors,' China's Rural Families Suffer," *New York Times*, March 14, 2001

Nourishing Traditions—The Cookbook That Challenges Politically Correct Nutrition and the Diet Dictocrats, Revised Second Edition, Sally Fallon and Mary G. Enig, Ph.D. New Trends Publishing, 1999

Malinow MR, et al, "Reduction of plasmahomocysteine levels by breakfast cereal fortified with folic acid in patients with coronary heart disease." *New England Journal of Medicine*, 1998

Nutritional Evaluation of Food Processing, 3rd. Ed., E. Karmas and R. S. Harris. Van Nostrand Reinhold, 1987

Modern Nutrition in Health and Disease, 8th Ed., M.E. Shils, J.A. Olson and M. Shike. Lea & Febiger, 1994

National Research Council. Recommended Dietary Allowances, 11th Ed. Washington D.C.: National Academy of Sciences, 1998

CHAPTER 4 — Vitamin C: The Missing Link to Good Health

Rath M, Pauling L, "A unified theory of human cardiovascular disease leading the way to

the abolition of this disease as a cause for human mortality." *Journal of Orthomolecular Medicine*, 1992

Stone I, "The genetic disease: *Hypoascorbemia.*" *Acta Geneticae Medicae et Gemellogogiae,* 1967

Stone I, "Studies of a Mammalian Enzyme System for Producing Evolutionary Evidence on Man." *American Journal of Physical Anthropology,* 1967

The Healing Factor: Vitamin C Against Disease, I. Stone. Grosset and Dunlap, New York, 1972

Verrax J, et al, "The association of vitamins C and K3 kills cancer cells primarily by autoschizis, a novel form of cell death: Basis for their potential use as coadjuvants in anticancer therapy," Invited Review, *European Journal of Medicinal Chemistry,* 2003

Gilloteaux J, et al, "Autoschizis: another cell death for cancer cells induced by oxidative stress." *Itailan Journal of Anat Embryol,* 2001

How to Live Longer and Feel Better, Linus Pauling. W.H. Freeman & Co, 1986

Patterson JC, "Capillary rupture with intimal haemorrhage in the causation of cerebral vascular lesions, *Arch Pathology,* 1940

Willis GC, "An experimental study of the intimal ground substance in atherosclerosis," *Canadian M.A. Journal,* 1953

De Nigris F, et al, "Beneficial effects of antioxidants and L-arginine on oxidation—sensitive gene expression and endothelial NO synthase activity at sites of disturbed shear stress," *Proceedings of the National Academy of Science,* e-published ahead of print. 2003

Heart Disease: A Textbook of Cardiovascular Medicine, E. Braunwald, Editor. W. B. Sanders & Co. Philadelphia, 2004

Veterinary Pathology, T.C. Jones, H.A. Smith. Lea and Febiger, 1958

The Fat Fallacy: The French Diet Secrets to Permanent Weight Loss, Dr. Will Clower. Perusal Press, 2003

Nourishing Traditions—The Cookbook That Challenges Politically Correct Nutrition and the Diet Dictocrats, Revised Second Edition, Sally Fallon and Mary G. Enig, Ph.D. New Trends Publishing, 1999 ("Everyone knows this is the Long Life Diet…" Elizabeth Rosenthal in the *New York Times.*)

Shah PK, "Plaque disruption and thrombosis: potential role of inflammation and infection," *Cardiology Review,* 2000

Romeo F, et al, "Role of infection in atherosclerosis and precipitation of acute cardiac events" *Progress in Inflammation Research,* 2001 (M.J. Parnham, Ed. Birkhauser Verlag, Basel, Switzerland)

Scannapieco F, et al, "Association of periodontal infections with atherosclerotic and pulmonary diseases," *Journal of Periodontal Research*, 1999

Sugar: Chemical, Biological and Nutritional Aspects of Sucrose, Edited by Yudkin, Edelman and Hough, Butterworth's, 1971

Sweet and Dangerous, John Yudkin. Peter H. Wyden, 1972

Ascorbate, The Science of Vitamin C, Dr. Steve Hickey PhD & Dr. Hilary Roberts PhD, LuLu Press, 2004

CHAPTER 5 — Sugar: Public Enemy Number One

"Junk Food, Food Junk," Allen Durning, printed in *World Watch* Sept./Oct. 1991

Fighting the Food Giants, Paul Stitt. Natural Press, 1980

Sweet and Dangerous, John Yudkin. Peter H. Wyden, New York, 1972

Excitotoxins:The Taste That Kills, R.L. Blaylock. Health Press, 1996

Ikonomidou C, et al, "Sensitivity of the developing rat brain to hypobaric/ischemic damage parallels sensitivity to N-Methyl-Asparate neurotoxicity." *Journal of Neuroscience*, 1989

Beck B, et al, "Effects of long term ingestion of aspartame on hypothalamic neuropeptide Y, plasma leptin and body weight gain and composition." *Physiology and Behavior*, 2002

Coulombe RA, et al, "Neurobiochemical alterations induced by the artificial sweetener aspartame (NutraSweet)." *Toxicology and Applied Pharmacology*, 1986

Olney JW, "Excitotoxins in foods." *Neurotoxicology*, 1994

Olney JW, et al, "Increasing Brain Tumor Rates: Is there a link to aspartame?" *Journal of Neuropathology and Experimental Neurology*, 1996

The Fat Fallacy, Dr. Will Clower, PhD. Three Rivers Press, 2002

For more on NutraSweet's 1981 approval by FDA, see: www.swankinturner.com/aspertame/hist.html

Tsang Wing-Sum, et al, "Determination of aspartame and its breakdown products in soft drinks by reverse-phase chromatography with UV detection." *Journal Agriculture and Food Chemistry*, 1985

Kaa-he-e, Its Nature and Properties, by Dr. Moises N. Bertoni. Paraguayan Scientific Analysis, December 1905.

The Stevia Story: A Tale of Incredible Sweetness & Intrigue, Donna Gates. Vital Health

Publishing, 2000

Rob McCaleb's quote comes from an article by Linda and Bill Vonvie, "Sinfully Sweet?"
in *New Age Journal*, Jan-Feb, 1996

Richard Adamson is quoted in an article by Thomas H. Burton and Betsy McKay, "Study Links Sugar-Sweetened Soft Drinks and Diabetes." *Wall St. Journal*

Read more about General Mills ad campaign targeted at children in the *Wall St. Journal*, Wednesday, June 22, 2005.

CHAPTER 6—Milk in America

For more on the mass production of milk, see www.realmilk.com

FAO database on internet: www.fao.org/StasticalDatabase/Food Balance Sheet Reports.

Fuchs NK, "Magnesium: A Key to Calcium Absorption." http://www.mgwater.com November, 2002

Abraham G, et al, "A total dietary program emphasizing magnesium instead of calcium. *Journal of Reproductive Medicine*, 1990

Misof BM et al, "Effect on bone and mineral metabolism in the mouse." *Calcified Tissue Institute*, 2003

Verslius RG, et al, "Prevalence of osteoporosis in post menopausal women in the Netherlands. *Tijdscher Geneesk*, 1999

Lau EM, et al, "Admission rates for hip fracture in Australia in the last decade." *Medical Journal of Australia*, 1993

Fujita T and Fukase M, "Comparison of osteoporosis and calcium intake in Japan and the United States." *Professional Society for the Exploration of Biological Medicine*, 1992/2000

Bauer RL, "Ethnic difference in the hip fracture: A reduced incidence in Mexican Americans." *American Journal of Epidemiology*, 1988

Kessenich CR, "Osteoporosis and African-American Women," *Women's Health Issues*, 2000

Xu Lu, et Al, "Very low rates of hip fracture in Beijing, People's Republic of China: The Beijing Osteoporosis Project." *American Journal of Epidemiology*, 1996

Ho SC, et al, "The Prevalence of osteoporosis in the Hong Kong female population." *Maturitas*, 1999

"Land, Water and Energy Versus the Ideal U.S. Population," published by the Negative Population Growth (NPG) Forum, a national membership organization founded in 1972 to alert citizens of the environmental consequences of overpopulation.

The Untold Story of Milk, Green Pastures, Contented Cows and Raw Dairy Foods, Ron Schmid, ND. New Trends Publishing, 2003

Epstein SS, "Unlabeled Milk from cows treated with biosynthetic growth hormones: a case of regulatory abdication." *International Journal of Health Services,* 1996

Rice DN, Bodman GR, "The Somatic Cell Count and Milk Quality." Cooperative Extension, Institute of Agriculture and Natural Resources, University of Nebraska-Lincoln web site, www.ianr.unl.edu/pubs/dairy/g1151.htm,

Gutnecht, Kurt, "Dire warnings about Johne's Disease—a wake up call for the Dairy Industry?" *Wisconsin Agriculturist,* December 2000. Access at www.moomilk.com/archive/nutrition-16.htm.

US Army Office of the Surgeon General: "Possible link between Johne's Disease and Crohn's Disease?" Article posted on a US Military Health Blog, www.hooah4health.com/environment/johnes.htm July 9, 2003

CHAPTER 7—The Great Soy Menace to Your Health

How to Live Longer and Feel Better, Linus Pauling. W.H.Freeman & Co., 1986

The Whole Soy Story—The Dark Side of America's Favorite Health Food, Kaayla T. Daniel, PhD, CCN. New Trends Publishing, 2007.

Levitt C, Yan L, Paull GL, Potter SM, *Solae LLC, Health Claim Petition: Soy Protein and the Reduced Risk of Certain Cancers.* Submitted to FDA, February 11, 2004, as reported in *The Whole Soy Story—The Dark Side of America's Favorite Health Food,* by Kaayla T. Daniel, PhD.

Mihagi Y, et al, "Trypsin inhibitor activity in commercial soybean products in Japan." *Journal of Nutritional Science Vitaminol,* 1997

The Book of Miso: Savory Soy Seasoning, William Shurtleff and Aikiko Aoyagi. Ten Speed Press, 2001

Golbitz, Peter, "Soyfoods Consumption in the United States and Worldwide, a Statistical Analysis." www.soyatech.com

"Chronology of Soymilk Worldwide: Part I, 220 AD to 1949," William Shurtleff. Special Exhibit, Museum of Soy, 2001, www.soydailyclub.com

"Crop Blight: Monsanto falls flat trying to sell Europe on bioengineered food. Its soybeans are safe, say trade officials, but public doesn't want to hear about it." Scott Killman and Helene Cooper. *Wall St. Journal*, May 11, 1999

"Group sows seeds of revolt against genetically altered foods in the US," Lucette Lagnado. *Wall St. Journal*, May 11, 1999

Masaharu Kawata, "Monsanto's Dangerous Logic as Seen in the Application Documents Submitted to the Health Ministry in Japan." *Third World Bio-safety Information Service*, July 28, 2003. www.organicconsumers.org

History of Soybeans and Soyfoods: Past, Present, and Future, William Shurtleff. Lafayette, CA. Soy Foods Center, 1983

For "Evaluation of the health aspects of soy protein isolates as food ingredients," 1979. SCOGS-101, Prepared for Bureau of Foods, Food and Drug Administration by the Life Sciences Research Office, FASEB, see *The Whole Soy Story: The Dark Side of America's Favorite Health Food* by Kaayla T. Daniel, PhD. New Trends Publishing, 2007

"Proposed Health Claim for Soy Protein-Containing Products and a Reduced Risk of Heart Disease." Petition submitted by Marshall McMarcus, Director Regulatory and Trade Affairs, Protein Technologies International, May 4, 1998

Fallon, Sally and Enig, Mary G, "Tragedy and Hype: The Third International Soy Symposium." *Nexus*, April-May, 2000

Letters to Documents Management Branch (H.F.A. 305), Food and Drug Administration quoting Section 403, by Valerie James. James writes the FDA it is not "authorized to regulate on anything other than the petition to the agency. That is, it cannot 'substitute' a variation on the claim and make a proposed (or actual) ruling on the substituted purpose." September 16, 1999.

Anderson JW, Johnstone BM, Cook-Newell ME, "Meta-analysis of the effects of soy protein intake on serum liquids." *New England Journal of Medicine*, 1995

Fitzpatrick M, "Soy formulas and the effects of isoflavones on the thyroid." *New Zealand Medical Journal*, 2000

Ishizuki Y, et al, "The effects on the thyroid gland of soybeans administered experimentally in healthy subjects." *Nippon Naibundi Gakkai Zasshi*, 1991. Translation by Japan Communication Service,

Wellington. Courtesy Valerie and Richard James.

Hirayama T, "Epidemiology of prostate cancer with special reference to the role of diet." *National Cancer Institute Monograph*, 1979

Nourishing Traditions, Sally Fallon and Mary Enig. New Trends Publishing, Second Edition, 1999

Sheehan DM, "Isoflavone content of breast milk and soy formulas: benefits and risks (letter)." *Clinical Chemistry,* 1997

Eklund G, Oskarsson A, "Exposure of cadmium from infant formulas and weaning foods." *Food Additives Contam*, 1999, 16, 12, 509-519

Dabeka RW, McKenzie AW, "Lead, cadmium and fluoride levels in milk and infant formulas in Canada." *Journal Association Of Analytical Chemistry*, 1987

Fomon SJ, Edstrand J, "Fluoride Intake by Infants." Journal of Public Health Dentistry, 1999

Silva M, Reynolds EC, "Fluoride content of infant formulae in Australia." *Australian Dentistry Journal*, 1996

Tran TT, et al, "Effect of high dietary manganese intake of neonatal rats on tissue mineral accumulation, striatal dopamine levels, and neurodevelopmental status." *Neurotoxicology*, 2002

Tran TT, et al, "Effects of neonatal dietary manganese exposure on brain dopamine levels and neurocognitive functions," *Neurotoxicology*, 2002

Stasny D, et al, "Manganese intake and serum manganese concentration of human milk-fed and formula fed infants." *American Journal of Clinical Nutrition*, 1984

Lonnerdal B, et al, "Iron, zinc, copper and manganese in infant formulas." *American Journal Diseased Children* 1983

"Lumen Foods adds infant warning to soymilk." PR Newswire via NewsEdge Corporation 6/18/01. www.soyatech.com

For more on Dr. Nightingales' warning about use of soymilks for formula, see www.uiuc.edu/archives/experts/utilization/1998a/0746.html.

FDA *Consumer Magazine*, September 1990, DHHS Publication 91-2236

Draft Report of the *Committee on Toxicity,* Working Group on Phytoestrogens, as presented in *The Whole Soy Story—The Dark Side of America's Favorite Health Food*, Kaayla T. Daniel, PhD. New Trends Publishing, 2007

Price KR et al, "Naturally occurring estrogens in foods: a review. *Food*

Additives Contam, 1985

For more on the warning that 100 grams of soy protein has as much estrogen as one contraceptive pill, see Bulletin from the Swiss Federal Health Service (*Bulletin de L'Office Federal de la Santa Publique*, no. 28, July 20, 1992). Proportional to bodyweight, an infant would receive a dose equal to three to five birth control pills daily.

Baskin, Laurence S. (Ed.) "Hypospadias and Genital Development." *Advances in Experimental Medicine and Biology*, Vol. 545. Kluwer Academic/Plenum Publishers, 2004

Giddens Herman, et al, "Secondary sexual characteristics and menses in young girls seen in office practice." Study from the *Pediatric Research in Office Settings Network*, 1997

Montague, Peter, Editorial: The Obscenity of Accelerated Child Development. *Ecologist*, 1993

Zacharias L and Wurtman RJ, "Age at menarche." *New England Journal of Medicine*. 1969. The article includes results reported in: Michaelson N, "Studies in physical development of Negroes. IV. Onset of puberty." *Am Journal Physical Anthropology, 1944.*

Huang AS, et al, "Characterization of the nonvolatile minor constituents responsible for the objectionable taste of defatted soybean flour." *Journal of Food Science, 47, 19*

For more on content and taste of soy products, see study by Arthur D. Little & Soytech showing soymilk falls short of taste standards. Business wire via NewsEdge Corporation. Posted 8/21/01. www.soyatech.com

"Benchmarking soymilk flavor: US Market 2001: new soymilk flavor study shows wide range in quality." Soyatech Press Release. Posted 06/18/01. www.soyatech.com

"TIAX's Center for Food Reformulation shows sugar levels in soymilk on the rise." August 13, 2003. www.thesoydaily.com

Wakabayashi K, et al "Food-derived mutagens and carcinogens. *Cancer Research*, 1992

Oishi K, et al, "A case-control study of prostatic cancer with reference to dietary habits." *Prostate*, 1998

Soy Smart Health: Discover the "Super Food" That Fights Breast Cancer, Heart Disease, Osteoporosis, Menopausal Discomforts, and Estrogen Dominance, Neil Solomon, Richard Passwater, Rita Elkins. Woodland Publishing, 2000

CHAPTER 8: How to Avoid Cancer

Doll R and Peto R, "The causes of cancer: Quantitative estimates of avoidable risks of
cancer in the United States today." *Journal of the National Cancer Institute*, 1981

Libby P, "Atherosclerosis: the new view." *Scientific American*, May, 2002

Virmani R, et al, "Inflammation in coronary atherosclerosis-pathological aspects." *Progress in Inflammation Research*, (M.J Parnham, Ed.) Birkhauser Verlag, Basel, Switzerland 2001

Schieffer B, and Drexler H, "Role of interleukins in relation to the rennin-angiotension-system in atherosclerosis." *Progression in Inflammation Research* (M.J. Parnham, Ed.) Birkhauser Verlag, Basel, Switzerland 2001

"Issues in a Nutshell: 'Pasture Based Cattle', San Francisco Farmer's Market." 2005, CUESA, www.cuesa.org

"None of Us Should Eat Extra Estrogen," *Los Angeles Times*, March 24, 1997

The Paleolithic Prescription, S. Boyd Eaton MD, Marjorie Shostak, and Melvin Konner MD, PhD. Harper Collins, 1988

Scotto and Blair, "Rigoni-Stern and Medical Statistics: A Nineteenth Century Approach to Cancer Research." *Journal of Historical Medicine and Allied Science*, 1969

Out of My Life and Thought, Dr. Albert Schweitzer. Henry Holt & Co., 1933, 1949

Dogteam Doctor: The Story of Dr. Romig, Eva Greenslit Anderson. Caxton Printer's Edition, 1943

Nutrition and Physical Degeneration, 6th Edition, Weston A. Price, DDS. Keats Publishing, 1939

Health in the 21st Century, Will Doctors Survive? Francisco Contreras, MD. Nutri Books Corp., 1997

Epstein SS, "American Cancer Society: The World's Wealthiest 'Non-Profit' Institution." *International Journal of Health Services* Vol. 29, No. 3, 1999

DiLorenzo T.J. "One Charity's Uneconomic War on Cancer." *Wall St. Journal*, March 15, 1999

Health is Your Birthright: How to Create the Health You Deserve, Ellen Tart-Jensen, PhD. Celestial Arts, 1997

Steven Gray and Ilan Brat, "Prostate Tests Draw New Questions." *Wall St. Journal,* January 10, 2006

David P. Hamilton, "Ex-Executive Backs Big Push to Get a Jump on Cancer." Wall St. Journal, 2006

Amy Dockser Marcus, "At 32, a Decision: Is Cancer Small Enough to Ignore?" *Wall St. Journal,* Dec. 20, 2004

Tara Parker-Pope, "Doctors Seek to Identify Which Patients can Avoid Prostate Cancer Treatment," *Wall St. Journal,* 2006

Anti-Oxidants: Powerful Guardians Against Disease and Illness, David Delson. Fast Facts Publications, 1996

"Cellular prostatic zinc concentration correlates inversely with the amount of prostatic enlargement." *Investigative Urology*,1969. As cited in *BPH (Benign Prostatic Hypertrophy) & Prostate Cancer*, Kurt W. Donsbach, D.C. N.D., PhD. The Rockland Corporation, 1994

Fahim MS et al, "Zinc treatment for the reduction of hyperplasia of the prostate."

Federal Proceedings, 1976

BPH (Benign Prostatic Hypertrophy) & Prostate Cancer, Kurt W. Donsbach, D.C. N.D., PhD. The Rockland Corporation, 1994

Herbal Insights and Reflections, Spring 1994 Brochure published by Kroeger Herb Products, Boulder, CO.

How to Get Well, Paavo O. Airola, ND, PhD. Health Plus Publishers, 1974

Roberta B. Ness, MD, MPH and Jane A. Cauley, PhD, "Antibiotics may increase breast cancer risk," *Journal of American Medical Association,* Feb. 18, 2004

The Untold Story of Milk: Green Pastures, Contented Cows and Raw Dairy Foods, Ron Schmid, ND. New Trends Publishing, 2003

Anatomy of an Illness, Norman Cousins. W.W. Norton & CO, 1979

CHAPTER 9—How To Lose Weight—All About Fasting

Rackis JJ, "Biologically active components." In *Soybeans: Chemistry and Technology,*

Allan K Smith and Sidney J. Circle, Eds. Avi, 1972

Johnson LA and Myers DJ, "Industrial uses for soybeans." In *Practical Handbook of Soybean Processing and Utilization*, David R. Erickson, Ed. AOCS Press, 1995

Shurtleff W and Aoyaki A, "History of Soybean Crushing: Soy Oil and Soybean Meal." In *History of Soybeans and Soyfoods: Past, Present and Future (Lafayette, CA. soyfoods Center)*, unpublished manuscript, as reported in *The Whole Soy Story—The Dark Side of America's Favorite Health Food*, Kaayla T. Daniel, PhD. New Trends Publishing, 2007

"Changes in Diet can Sometimes Lead to Hair Loss," Tara Parker-Pope. *Wall St. Journal*, Sept. 13, 2005

Poole, Robert M., "The Incredible Machine," National Geographic Society Book Service, 1986.

Liver Disease and Gallstones, The Facts, Johnson, Alan G. and Triger, David R. Oxford University Press, New York, 1987

How to Live Longer and Feel Better, Linus Pauling, W.H. Freeman & Co., 1986

The Fasting Path: The Way to Spiritual, Physical and Emotional Enlightenment, Stephen Harrod Buhner, Avery Press, 2003

NIGGER, Dick Gregory. Buccaneer Books 1993

The Miracle of Fasting: Proven Throughout History for Physical, Mental and Spiritual Rejuvenation by Paul C. Bragg. Bragg Live Foods, 1999

Note about whale's feeding patterns: Due to increased monitoring and whale watching, it is now known that gray whales do occasionally feed, both in Scammons Lagoon in Baja while giving birth and occasionally as they journey north. Two juvenile gray whales once spent an entire summer feeding at San Miguel Island, offshore from Santa Barbara and were often observed feeding in shallow waters.

CHAPTER 10: The Business of Food—
How Mass Produced Food Can Make You Sick and Fat

What Doctors Don't Tell You, Lynn McTaggart. HarperCollins, 2005

"The Good Egg," Cheryl Long and Umut Newbury. *Mother Earth News*, August/September 2005

The Omega Diet, Artemis Simopoulos. Harper Collins, 1988

Mad Cowboy: Plain Truth from the Cattle Rancher Who Won't Eat Meat, Howard F. Lyman and Glen Merzer. Scribner, 1998

Cancer—Step Outside the Box, Ty M. Bollinger. Infinity 510 Partners, 2006

Waste of the West, Lynn Jacobs. Arizona Lithographers, 1981

World News Network BP Statistical Review of World Energy: Total Oil

consumption of 75,291,00 barrels/day in 2001. OECD countries
consumed 47,471,000 barrels a day in 2001.
Statistics on how much oil is used to grow corn from "When a Crop
Becomes King," by Michael Pollan. *New York Times*, July 19, 2002.
Fighting the Food Giants, Paul Stitt. Nature Press, 1980

CHAPTER 11: Food That's Good For You to Eat

"Physicians Health Study," *Current Atherosclerosis Reports*, 1999
Tara Parker-Pope, "Want Fat With That? A Surprising Way to Make
Vegetables More
Nutritious." *Wall Street Journal,* August 9, 2006
Nutrition and Physical Degeneration, Weston A. Price, DDS. Keats Press,
1939